PELVIC PAIN EXPLAINED

PELVIC PAIN EXPLAINED

What You Need to Know

Stephanie A. Prendergast and Elizabeth H. Rummer

ROWMAN & LITTLEFIELD
Lanham • Boulder • New York • London

Published by Rowman & Littlefield
A wholly owned subsidary of
The Rowman & Littlefield Publishing Group, Inc.
4501 Forbes Boulevard, Suite 200, Lanham, Maryland 20706
www.rowman.com

Unit A, Whitacre Mews, 26-34 Stannary Street, London SE11 4AB

British Library Cataloguing in Publication Information Available

Library of Congress Cataloging-in-Publication Data

The hardback edition of this book was previously cataloged by the Library of
Congress as follows:

Prendergast, Stephanie A., 1976–
Pelvic pain explained : what you need to know / Stephanie A. Prendergast and
Elizabeth H. Akincilar.
pages cm
Includes bibliographical references and index.
ISBN 978-1-4422-4831-1 (cloth : alk. paper) — ISBN 978-1-4422-4832-8
(electronic) — 978-0-8108-9591-1 (paperback)
1. Pelvic floor—Diseases. 2. Pelvic floor—Diseases—Treatment. I. Akincilar,
Elizabeth H., 1976– II. Title.
RG482.P74 2016
617.5'5—dc23
2015024826

♾™ The paper used in this publication meets the minimum requirements
of American National Standard for Information Sciences—Permanence of
Paper for Printed Library Materials, ANSI/NISO Z39.48-1992.

Printed in the United States of America

CONTENTS

FOREWORD

If you suffer with pelvic pain, you need to read this book. Maybe several times. If you have a loved one with pelvic pain, both of you need to read this book. If you are a clinician who cares for patients with pelvic pain, you need to read this book. It is a down-to-earth, clearly written book that will educate and guide you in managing and relieving persistent pelvic pain.[1]

As you will learn when you read *Pelvic Pain Explained*, persistent pelvic pain is a common condition that affects people of every race, gender, socioeconomic group, and profession—it is a ubiquitous condition of all humans. It is as common as asthma, migraine, and low back pain. As is the case for all persistent pain conditions, it affects all aspects of the sufferer's life, but because of the location in the pelvis, it usually affects sexuality and intimacy far more than is the case with other pain conditions. For that reason, Liz and Stephanie devote a whole chapter to sex and pelvic pain.

Some may be concerned that the authors of this book are physical therapists, not physicians. You should not be. I am a physician who spent most of my clinical and academic career dedicated to caring for patients with persistent pelvic pain, doing research on pelvic pain, and teaching others about pelvic pain. I was one of the three founders of the International Pelvic Pain Society. This society has grown to be a premier organization dedicated to teaching about and care of patients with pelvic pain. It has more members who are physical therapists than physicians. When you read this book, you will have a clear understanding of why that is the case. I learned very early in my career that persistent pelvic pain, for all intents and purposes, always involves the musculoskeletal system, either as a primary or a secondary generator of pain. Physical therapists are ideal clinicians to deal with the musculoskeletal sources of pelvic pain, even when other bodily systems are also involved. They should always be part of the treatment team. So it is very appropriate that two physical therapists wrote *Pelvic Pain Explained*.

Stephanie and Liz are ideal physical therapists to be authors of this book. As they explain in their introduction, they have 30 years of combined experience both treating patients and educating providers. They have worked hard in their careers not only educating others, but also educating themselves. They have treated thousands of patients, male and female, and have a deep understanding of the approach to treatment that is needed if it is to be successful. This includes the strong involvement of the patient. Thus, they devote the whole third segment of their book to what the patient must do to stop being a patient, and return to being a "person." One of the most consistent frustrations during my 30 years treating women with persistent pelvic pain was the realization that if I was working harder than my patient to try to make her better, then we were both doomed to failure. Liz and Stephanie tell you in *Pelvic Pain Explained* what you need to do so that will not happen to you and your health care team. Additionally, they will help you navigate the complexities of our health care systems so you can find a team of clinicians that can educate, treat, and guide you to relieving your pain. Persistent pelvic pain is a complicated malady, and you will find that no one single provider will be able to help with you all the aspects of education and treatment that you will need.

So read this book if you are a patient, have a loved one, or are a clinician dealing with pelvic pain. Let it help you on your path to being well and pain-free, or having your loved one or your patient be pain-free.

Fred M. Howard, M.S., M.D.
Chairman of the Board
International Pelvic Pain Society
Professor Emeritus of Obstetrics and Gynecology
University of Rochester School of Medicine and Dentistry
St. John
United States Virgin Islands

ACKNOWLEDGMENTS

Thank you to Bonnie Bauman whom without her initiation, contributions, and support this book would not have been written. Thank you to Maria Lluberes for her wonderful illustrations.

We would like to thank the thousands of patients that trusted us with their health, providing us with the knowledge, experience, and passion to write this book. We would like to give a special thank you to Rhonda Kotarinos who paved the way for us as well as other physical therapists in this field. As the field grew, the International Pelvic Pain Society (IPPS) helped us further our education but also provided us with our first platform for teaching. We know this book would not have happened without each other and our extremely committed PHRC team. And, finally, we thank our supportive friends and family who are always there through our joys and successes.

INTRODUCTION

Anyone with persistent pelvic pain knows that getting on the right treatment path is often half the battle. The main reason for this is that persistent pain in general is a poorly understood medical condition compared to other diagnoses. So at the end of the day, many people with pelvic pain—while in the throes of dealing with symptoms that wreak havoc on their daily lives—are struggling to find answers. They're not alone in their frustration. Medical providers are often equally at a loss as they find themselves up against a lack of available research and education. The good news is that in recent years, a growing group of physicians, pelvic floor physical therapists, and psychologists are becoming actively involved in the research and management of pelvic pain syndromes. But while the landscape for treatment *is* improving, for many people with pelvic pain, getting a correct diagnosis and the appropriate treatment continues to be an uphill battle. We wrote this book to address that challenge. The purpose of this book is to act as a guide for patients and providers as they navigate the many complexities associated with the pelvic pain treatment process. As clinicians, we have a combined 30 years of experience both treating patients and educating providers. Over the years we've treated thousands of patients from one end of the pelvic pain spectrum to the other. As a result, we've learned what works (and what doesn't) in successfully treating pelvic pain. In the pages of this book we share that knowledge.

WHAT IS THIS BOOK ABOUT?

At its heart, *Pelvic Pain Explained* is an exploration of pelvic pain from how patients get it to the challenges both patients and providers face throughout the treatment process to a discussion of the impact that an "invisible" condition has on a patient's life and relationships, and much more. Patients will walk away from this book with a complete understanding of pelvic pain, from how it occurs to the variety of symptoms associated with it to how the impairments and contributing factors that are causing their symptoms are uncovered and treated. In addition, the book will provide patients with an understanding of all the current treatment options available to them. Those who develop pelvic pain can find the path to treatment frustrating and unsuccessful, oftentimes because they're attempting to work within the framework of recovery that they're used to; one in which they go to the doctor, maybe have some diagnostic testing done, then get a very specific diagnosis that dictates a very specific mode of treatment. This simply is not the path to recovery from pelvic pain. Pelvic pain is a health issue that often crosses the borders between medical disciplines because of the many different systems that can be involved. Gynecologists, urologists, gastroenterologists, orthopedists, pain management specialists, psychologists, and acupuncturists, among others, all have a role in treating the pelvic floor. In addition, for recovery to occur, the patient must be an active participant in the treatment process. This book provides patients with the guidance they need to navigate this unfamiliar treatment framework, thus placing them on the right path to recovery. For providers, the book demystifies pelvic pain. In addition, it contains information that will help them troubleshoot in situations where patients either cannot tolerate or are unresponsive to a particular treatment approach. As the information in these pages will prove, when a particular treatment doesn't work, another option exists.

The book is organized into three parts. The goal of the first part of the book is to give readers an overview of pelvic pain. Toward that end, the chapters in this section discuss the symptoms, causes, and factors that contribute to pelvic pain as well as explain the role of the neuromuscular system in the condition. Part II of the book lays out the path to recovery from pelvic pain. This part of the book provides guidance on how patients can assemble the best team of providers, takes readers through the pelvic pain PT process, and provides a complete overview of the many different treatment options available for the condition. In addition, part II covers pelvic pain–related issues concerning pregnancy and sexual health. Part III places patients in the driver's seat of their recovery by giving them actionable information. At-home self-treatment strategies, tips on communicating with providers and staying fit while in recovery, as well as practical tips for day-to-day living are among the topics covered in this section.

HOW WILL THIS BOOK HELP ME THROUGH TREATMENT?

This book aims to provide a stepping-off point for those with pelvic pain to begin to navigate the treatment process. Toward that end, it provides answers to the many questions they have as they stand on the threshold of their treatment journey, such as: *How did I get pelvic pain? What is the best way to treat pelvic pain? What are my treatment options? How do I find qualified and knowledgeable providers? How do I navigate day-to-day life with pelvic pain?* In addition, it guides patients through the many complexities that arise during the treatment and recovery process, such as what to do when treatments don't work; how to improve communication with medical providers; how to remain calm during a flare; and how to cope with the many emotional issues that crop up during the recovery process, among many others. Our main intention in writing this book is to streamline the treatment process for both patients and providers. Oftentimes patients fall into treatment traps, such as wasting time and money on unnecessary procedures that may make their condition worse. Just as often, they don't fully understand the treatment modalities they sign up for, so they're not compliant, and for that reason, they don't get better. For all of these reasons, in this book we don't just present information about pelvic pain; we combine it with the comprehensive assessment skills we've gained from our own experience as clinicians and educators. So by reading it, both patients and providers are not just informing themselves about pelvic pain, they're also beginning to think critically about the issues that surround the treatment process, thus better arming themselves for decision making along the way.

CAN READING THIS BOOK HELP ME GET BETTER?

Yes. For one thing, research shows that educating patients about the physiology behind their symptoms reduces stress, and in turn that reduces pain.[1] The information in this book will demystify pelvic pain for readers so they will have less stress and anxiety surrounding their pain. Also, the book will help patients get better by helping them to navigate the pelvic pain treatment process. It will help direct them to the right providers, allow them to make educated treatment choices, alert them to the right questions to ask, and, in general, enable them to be unintimidated by the treatment process. At the end of the day, all of this *will* help patients get better.

WHY DID PTS WRITE THIS BOOK?

Physical therapy is becoming the standout of the new interdisciplinary treatment approach to persistent pain. In fact, in her best-selling book on persistent pain, *The Pain Chronicles*, author Melanie Thernstrom advises readers to commit to giving PT a try. "Truly, if you take any advice from this book, take this one," she writes. And *New York Times* author Barry Meier, in his controversial article "The Problem with Pain Pills," passes along similar advice. PT, along with an interdisciplinary treatment plan, is the way to go, he writes. And to further validate the central role that PT now plays in the treatment of persistent pain, lawmakers in all 50 states and the District of Columbia have some form of "direct access" law in place, allowing patients to have direct access to PTs without a physician referral or prescription. This emphasis on PT is especially relevant when treating pelvic pain. That's because PT is a main line of treatment for the majority of pelvic pain patients. Therefore, it makes sense for *the* definitive book on navigating pelvic pain to be written by PTs.

When we met each other a decade ago, we instantly bonded over our shared passion for helping people with pelvic pain. Spurred on by our desire to improve the standard of care for this patient population, we ultimately partnered up and opened our physical therapy practice, the Pelvic Health and Rehabilitation Center (PHRC). From the outset, our goal with PHRC was to improve the standard of care for pelvic pain treatment. At this point, we believe we have developed a successful treatment model, one that stresses an interdisciplinary approach to treatment, and we're looking forward to sharing it in these pages.

All our best,
Stephanie and Liz

I

Pelvic Pain: A Road Map

I

PELVIC PAIN 101

Ben, age 31, a competitive cyclist, has been suffering from penile, scrotal, and perineal pain for nearly eight months. After the birth of her second baby, Holly, 28, can no longer have sex with her husband without experiencing severe vaginal pain. Annie, a 20-year-old college student, has been forced to take a semester off from school due to the intense vestibular burning she developed after a fall onto her tailbone. Paul, a high-powered attorney in his mid-forties, who spends countless hours sitting at a desk or on an airplane, has been suffering from anal and sit bone pain for nearly a year. Shortly after undergoing a hysterectomy, Veronica, 65, developed vulvar burning and clitoral pain.

This is a cross section of the millions of men and women dealing with pelvic pain in the United States. Most people don't even know they have a pelvic floor until they experience pain or dysfunction. For this reason, we decided that the best way to begin our task of explaining pelvic pain was with a chapter that explored the basics of this pain syndrome. Toward that end, we begin the chapter with an overview of the pelvic floor and its functions. Next, we move to a general explanation of the causes and symptoms of pelvic pain. Lastly, we wrap up with a discussion of the challenges involved for patients seeking treatment as well as an explanation of what we consider to be the best approach to treating pelvic pain.

WHAT IS MY PELVIC FLOOR FOR?

The pelvic floor is a hammock-like group of 14 thin muscles intertwined with nerves and surrounded by connective tissue that supports the abdominal organs while playing a key role in urinary, bowel, and sexual function as well as postural support. When you consider the many ordinary (and extraordinary) tasks the pelvic floor plays a role in—childbirth, sex, bowel movements, urination, continence, sitting, walking—it's difficult to understand why it's such an underrecognized part of our human anatomy!

PELVIC PAIN CAUSES

Now that you have a basic understanding of what the pelvic floor is, let's discuss what can go wrong with this swath of muscles, nerves, and

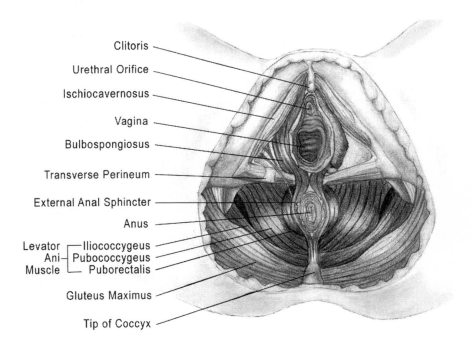

Figure 1.1.   Female pelvic floor muscles and perineum. *Source: Pelvic Health and Rehabilitation Center*

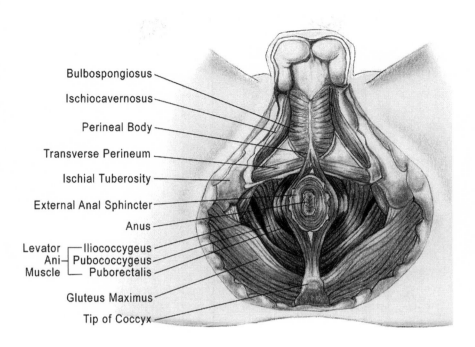

Bulbospongiosus

Ischiocavernosus

Perineal Body

Transverse Perineum

Ischial Tuberosity

External Anal Sphincter

Anus

Levator ⎡ Iliococcygeus
Ani ⎨ Pubococcygeus
Muscle ⎣ Puborectalis

Gluteus Maximus

Tip of Coccyx

Figure 1.2. **Male pelvic floor muscles and perineum.** *Source: Pelvic Health and Rehabilitation Center*

connective tissue to cause pelvic pain. In general, too-tight pelvic floor muscles, inflamed nerves of the pelvic floor, and/or restricted connective tissue are what ultimately will cause pelvic pain and urinary, bowel, and/or sexual dysfunction. *But how do these impairments occur?* The muscles, nerves, and connective tissue of the pelvic floor can become impaired in a number of ways. For example, childbirth; straining due to constipation; an injury, such as a fall on the tailbone; or repetitive activity, such as prolonged sitting, horseback riding, or cycling, can all lead to the development of a pelvic pain syndrome. In addition, any disease of the urinary, bowel, or reproductive systems, such as frequent urinary tract or yeast infections, bacterial prostatitis, or endometriosis can be the cause. More often than not, however, a combination of factors contributes to a patient's pain. Plus, it's common for symptoms to manifest after years of buildup with one incident serving as the proverbial "straw that broke the camel's back." For instance, a man works as a cashier at a grocery store, a job that requires him to repetitively rotate to the left as he scans groceries. As a result of this repetitive movement, the muscles on the left side of his body become tighter than those on the right. He then joins a gym to work out with the goal of becoming a better snowboarder. During his workouts he begins to do several sets of squats and sit-ups, which recruit the muscles on his right and left sides equally, but because the muscles on his left side are tighter from his job and therefore more vulnerable to injury, left abdominal trigger points develop. (A "trigger point" is a small, taut patch of involuntarily contracted muscle fibers within a muscle that can cause pain.) These trigger points begin to refer pain to the tip of his penis and perineum while he's working out at the gym. Finally, he falls on his tailbone several times snowboarding, so his penile and perineum pain becomes constant.

COMMON SYMPTOMS

Now that you have a general understanding of what causes pelvic pain, let's take a look at some of the more common symptoms associated with the condition. (This list is not meant to be definitive.)

In men symptoms may include:

- penile/scrotal/perineal or anal pain
- post-ejaculatory pain
- erectile dysfunction
- tailbone pain
- pain with sitting
- pain with exercise
- pain with urination, urinary urgency, frequency, hesitancy, and burning
- decreased force of urine stream
- constipation

In women symptoms can include:

- vulvar, vaginal, clitoral, perineal, or anal pain
- pain with sexual intercourse
- pain following sex
- interlabial, vulvar, or genital itching
- painful urination, urinary hesitancy, urgency, and/or frequency

- abdominal and groin pain
- sacroiliac joint pain/instability
- constipation
- painful periods
- pain with sitting
- pain with exercise

DIAGNOSIS AND TREATMENT CHALLENGES

Why is it so challenging to get a proper diagnosis and treatment for pelvic pain?

The answer to this question is multilayered. For one thing, persistent pain, which is commonly defined as pain that continues after tissue has healed, is poorly understood compared to other diagnoses. To be sure, until recently, clinical treatment for pain existed under the assumption that pain was a symptom of an underlying disease or trauma. The theory was that if you treated the underlying disease, the pain would go away. However, with persistent pain it often doesn't happen that way. Now researchers understand that pain in and of itself can be a diagnosis, and that left untreated, it has the potential to rewrite the central nervous system, causing changes to the brain and spinal cord, which can cause pain in the absence of an underlying cause. This represents a profound transformation in how those with persistent pain are evaluated. And it's only just in the past few years that it's trickled down into the treatment of pelvic pain.

Couple this with the fact that the treatment of pelvic pain diverges widely from the treatment of most medical conditions. Typically, when you have a medical problem, you go to the doctor, who perhaps runs a few tests, and then from there you get a diagnosis and treatment— usually some sort of medication. The diagnosis and treatment of pelvic pain simply does not work this way. For one thing, with pelvic pain, a "diagnosis" does not dictate treatment. Typically, pelvic pain ends up being a diagnosis of exclusion whereby other pathologies, such as an infection, must first be ruled out, and when symptoms persist, the patient is then given a descriptor diagnosis, such as "vulvodynia," which simply means "pain in the vulva." A second example is "interstitial cystitis/painful bladder syndrome" or "pudendal neuralgia," meaning pain in the bladder and the pudendal nerve distribution respectively. When a patient is given any one of these descriptor diagnoses, they're often confused and frustrated, mainly because none of them have specific, one-size-fits-all treatment protocols. *So if a diagnosis does not dictate treatment, what does?* What *does* dictate treatment for pelvic pain are the specific neurological, musculoskeletal, and psychological impairments that are uncovered and determined to be involved in a patient's symptoms. As already mentioned, pelvic pain is rarely caused by just one issue. Rather, more often than not, it's caused by a combination of factors, including impairments of the pelvic floor muscles, the central and peripheral nervous systems, and even behavioral issues, like poor posture or "holding in" one's urine. Therefore, a successful treatment approach involves identifying and treating all the different impairments contributing to a patient's symptoms. These impairments might be found in the muscles, joints, nerves, or connective tissue of the pelvic floor and girdle and/or the pelvic organs and the derma of the genitals. So we're not just talking about that hammock of 14 muscles described above. Therefore, the best course of action is to identify all the impairments that contribute to a patient's pelvic pain, and then treat each and every one of them individually while collectively treating the patient as a whole. But while a diagnosis does not dictate treatment for pelvic pain, oftentimes getting a specific diagnosis/diagnoses is necessary to work within our managed health care system. Take the point made by one of the readers of our blog:

> I've been given multiple diagnoses, and at least with the names, I'm getting treatment. For me, the different names to what is happening to my body do not matter except that the multiple doctors, PTs, etc. seem to treat just their specialty condition and without a name, it won't be treated. I strongly think that much of this is because our medical system is fragmented into so many specialties that don't interact, just refer. Now, I'm getting excellent care from my ob/gyn, pain doctor, gastroenterologist, and PT, but I wouldn't be getting treatment approved by our health insurance without a diagnosis, so for me the diagnosis equals treatment. Having a diagnosis seems to be a necessary evil in our fragmented, broken healthcare system.

Another departure from how most medical conditions are treated is that for the most part, a pelvic floor physical therapist will play the largest role in treating the impairments causing a patient's pain. That's because typically, those impairments are neuromuscular in nature, and physical therapy is the medical discipline that specializes in treating the neuromuscular system. So the typical scenario where patient visits doctor/patient gets diagnosis and treatment from doctor/patient gets well does not play out when it comes to pelvic pain.

The good news is that in just under a decade, tremendous strides have been made in the diagnosis and treatment of pelvic pain. For one thing, PTs have taken a solid leadership role in figuring out how to treat the condition. In addition, both physicians and PTs have embraced pelvic pain as a research topic. Also validating is the fact that at the time of this book's writing, a major initiative to improve the research and treatment of persistent pain includes pelvic pain as one of more than a dozen chronic pain syndromes that need an improved treatment approach.[1] Having solely treated the pelvic floor for more than 15 years, we understand the challenges involved with a pelvic pain diagnosis and treatment. We also know that it's possible for patients to navigate the current treatment landscape to get positive results. We see it every day in our clinics! And that's in essence what this book is about. After successfully treating thousands of patients, we know how to work within the current treatment landscape to get the best results.

PELVIC PAIN "DIAGNOSES"

While a diagnosis *should not* dictate treatment for pelvic pain, some diagnoses are *associated* with pelvic pain. Some of these diagnoses, such as endometriosis and interstitial cystitis, are disease processes where pelvic pain is a symptom. Others, such as pudendal neuralgia or vestibulodynia, fall under the category of "descriptor" diagnoses that we mentioned above and simply convey that pain is associated with a particular part of the body. We've provided a complete list of these diagnoses in the following list.

- vulvodynia, "primary/secondary" or "provoked/unprovoked": pain in the vulva
- dyspareunia: pain with sexual intercourse
- clitorodynia/genital pain: pain of the clitoris, genitalia
- penile pain
- anal pain
- perineum pain
- coccydynia: tailbone pain
- dysorgasmia: pain with orgasm
- pudendal neuralgia: pain in the distribution of the pudendal nerve
- vestibulodynia: pain of the vestibule
- vaginismus: severe pain upon attempted vaginal penetration or inability to achieve vaginal penetration
- orchialgia: pain in the testes

A BIOPSYCHOSOCIAL APPROACH TO TREATMENT

More and more, the medical community is moving toward treating the whole patient under a biopsychosocial model of care. Basically, this approach to medicine takes biological, psychological (thoughts, emotions, and behaviors), and social (socioeconomic and cultural) factors into consideration when treating a patient. We believe that a biopsychosocial model is the best approach to treating pelvic pain, and the way to put this model into practice is by taking an interdisciplinary treatment approach to treatment where all necessary medical disciplines are involved in a patient's recovery. Here's the reality: pelvic pain can cover many different systems of the body, including the musculoskeletal system, the urinary system, the reproductive system, the gastrointestinal (GI) system, the nervous system, and the endocrine system (hormones). On top of that, many of these systems have to be approached from different angles to successfully treat patients. For example, a patient who is having constipation issues may need to see a GI doctor, a nutritionist, and a PT to effectively treat his/her constipation. The GI doctor would rule out or treat any issues having to do with the patient's organs, a nutritionist might be needed to alter the patient's diet, and the PT will treat muscle dysfunction. So because pelvic pain can span so many different specialties in medicine, one lone specialty can't sufficiently evaluate and treat a complex pelvic pain case. The expertise of providers across disciplines is often required to effectively treat these cases. Gynecologists, urologists, gastroenterologists, orthopedists, pain management specialists, physical therapists, psychologists, and acupuncturists, among others, are all providers that have a role to play in treating pelvic pain syndromes.

THE ROLE OF THE PT IN TREATING PELVIC PAIN

The majority of pelvic pain cases will involve some kind of neuromuscular problem—a problem with the muscles, nerves, and connective tissue of the pelvic floor and adjacent areas. A PT is the medical provider who has the best understanding of these issues, and is therefore best equipped to treat them. Therefore, as mentioned above, a pelvic floor PT is going to play the largest role in treating a pelvic pain syndrome. But *what exactly is that role?*

In addition to uncovering and treating whatever neuromuscular impairments are driving a patient's symptoms, we believe that the best-case scenario is for the PT to take on the role of coordinator/facilitator of an interdisciplinary treatment plan, acting as a sort of patient "case manager." Here's why: an interdisciplinary treatment approach works best when one provider takes on the job of coordinating a patient's overall treatment plan. And with pelvic pain, it makes sense for the PT to take on the role of facilitator because number one, he/she will be spending the most time with the patient, and number two, he/she will be playing a major role in uncovering the patient's impairments. In our role as treatment facilitators, we not only uncover and treat whatever neuromuscular impairments exist, we also work with patients to figure out what other systems might be involved with their pain. If other systems do play a role, we help to get patients to the appropriate provider, acting as liaison with the assembled treatment team. We recognize that this puts a lot of responsibility onto PTs. To be sure, it's a big time commitment. But what we've observed in our practice is that if you want to successfully treat a person with pelvic pain, at the end of the day, it's what works.

In addition to facilitating a patient's interdisciplinary treatment plan, a PT often plays another, albeit less formal, role in treatment. While we're not psychologists and should never cross that line, the treatment we provide our patients has an emotional support component. Because we are often the provider who will spend the most time with patients, they have the opportunity to talk things through with us, to expose their fears and frustrations. Patients often apologize during their treatment session for "dumping" on us. Our response is always, "No apologies! That's what we're here for." As PTs, we work to encourage our patients and give them positive feedback throughout the recovery process. Sometimes this means giving them a nudge to go further in their recovery. For example, we may advise them to seek out other treatments, try intercourse for the first time after a break, or even to sit for 10 minutes longer than usual. So oftentimes a PT takes on the role of cheerleader during what can be a long treatment process.

JESSICA'S STORY

Since as far back as I can remember, I had on-and-off vestibule pain. In addition, all my life I've had bouts of constipation and hypermobile joints, meaning I am overly flexible (not a good thing). These are all factors that likely helped pave the way for my pelvic pain. One day when I was in my mid-twenties, I got a urinary tract infection that kicked off a downward spiral of constant vestibule and vaginal pain. That's when my search for answers began. Along the way, a urologist prescribed endless rounds of antibiotics. I underwent a cystoscopy, which is basically a bladder scope (ouch!), received an interstitial cystitis (IC) diagnosis, and got several more opinions from a variety of different doctors—a few of which concluded that my pain was caused by "stress." I read articles that convinced me that my symptoms were caused by "too much acid in my body" or "chronic yeast." These revelations resulted in some very extreme diets, including a "yeast cleanse." When all else failed, I spent hundreds of dollars on supplements, not because I necessarily thought they would help, but because I needed something proactive to do. Finally, months into my pain, I read about pelvic pain PT online, made an appointment to see Liz at PHRC, and started down the road to recovery. I won't lie and tell you that that road was an easy one. On the contrary, the ups and downs were crazy making. Along the way, I developed intense pain and fatigue. My joints even stopped working. I did nothing but lie around with my cat, go to doctor and PT appointments, and try my best to dress and feed myself. I had to take medical leave from school and work. I went on opiate painkillers, among other medications, including an antidepressant. I learned that chronic pain is a breeding ground for depression. It took about seven months of weekly PT for me to begin to feel better, and reach a turning point in my recovery. During my sessions with Liz, she worked internally on my tight pelvic floor, which she said was riddled with trigger points. In addition, she worked externally on my abdomen, thighs, and hips, where she found connective tissue restrictions. Besides my regular PT sessions, ice and heat helped, sitting on a cushion and not sitting too much helped, and using a foam roller to loosen tight muscles in my back and legs also helped.

It took about a year and a half of weekly PT for me to fully heal. Today, my vestibule and vaginal pain are completely gone. I have pain-free sex and normal orgasms. I can do any activity I want to and not experience pain. I wear underwear and jeans. (I wore wrap skirts with no underwear for more than a year.) And thanks to the education I received in PT, I am also super-aware of when and where I clench. I've learned that when I clench my abs, which I tend to do when I'm anxious or stressed, I feel pain in my pelvic floor. Therefore, deep breathing and relaxation exercises are a must for me during any stressful situation. I don't do yoga or sit-ups because they tense up my pelvic floor and abdomen. I bought an expensive office chair that I'll sit in for the rest of my working life. I no longer have the chronic fatigue (I was sleeping for more than 16 hours at a time at my worst). These days, I just think of myself as similar to someone with a bad back who shouldn't lift heavy things or overdo it. Lastly, I no longer wake up in the morning and think about pain. Instead, I think about what I'm going to eat that day (I love to eat!), who I'm going to see, and what I'm going to do. If you're in the midst of this condition, know that there is a way out, and as much as possible, have compassion for yourself. You're going through something hard, but you will get better.

CONCLUSION

In this chapter we've opened the door to the complex topic that is pelvic pain by taking a look at the basic anatomy of the pelvic floor, the causes of pelvic pain, and the many symptoms associated with the diagnosis. In addition, we've delved into the challenges involved with getting the appropriate treatment as well as what exactly constitutes that treatment. In the next chapter, we go into more detail about the factors that contribute to pelvic pain with the goal of answering a question that we get on a daily basis from patients: *"How did I get this?"*

HOW COMMON IS PELVIC PAIN IN THE UNITED STATES?

Pelvic pain is every bit as common as back pain in the United States.[1] A look at the statistics shows just how common the condition is:

- Twenty percent of women will suffer from pelvic pain at some point in their lives.[2]
- Vulvodynia affects up to 16% of all women.[3]
- The estimated annual economic burden of vulvodynia in the United States is $31 billion to $72 billion.[4]
- Prostatitis is the third most common diagnosis of men under 50 presented to urologists annually, and 90% to 95% of all "prostatitis" diagnoses are actually male pelvic pain, showing the overdiagnosis of actual prostatitis and the underdiagnosis of male pelvic pain.[5]
- Up to 2 million *men* in the United States meet the diagnostic definition for persistent pelvic pain.[6]
- Chronic pelvic pain accounts for 10% of all visits to the gynecologist.[7]
- One in four women experience chronic vulvar pain (a symptom of pelvic pain) at some point in their lives.[8]
- Roughly 60% of sexually active women will suffer from painful sex at some point in their lives.[9]

- In a normal pregnancy, 13% to 36% of first-time moms show severe levator ani injury, one cause of postpartum pelvic floor dysfunction.[10]
- Pelvic girdle pain (a major cause of pelvic pain in pregnancy) occurs in 20% of pregnant women; for an estimated 7% to 8%, it results in severe disability.[11]
- Twenty-four percent of women have pain with intercourse 18 months after giving birth.[12]

Notes

1. KT Zondervan et al., "Prevalence and Incidence of Chronic Pelvic Pain in Primary Care: Evidence from a National General Practice Database," *Journal of Obstetrics and Gynecology* 106 (1999): 1149–1155.

2. G Apte et al., "Chronic Female Pelvic Pain: Part I: Clinical Pathoanatomy and Examination of the Pelvic Region," *Pain Practice* 12 (2012): 88–110.

3. *Ibid.*

4. LA Sadownik, "Etiology, Diagnosis, and Clinical Management of Vulvodynia," *International Journal of Women's Health* 6 (2014): 437–449.

5. J Bergman and S Zeitlin, "Prostatitis and Chronic Prostatitis/Chronic Pelvic Pain Syndrome," *Expert Review of Neurotherapeutics* 7 (2007): 301–307.

6. G Habermacher, J Chason, and A Schaeffer, "Chronic Prostatitis/Chronic Pelvic Pain Syndrome," *Annual Review of Medicine* 57 (2006): 195–206.

7. Gyang et al., "Musculoskeletal Causes of Chronic Pelvic Pain: What Every Gynecologist Should Know," *American College of Obstetrics and Gynecology* 121 (2013): 645–650.

8. *Ibid.*

9. *Ibid.*

10. N Schwertner-Tiepelmann et al., "Obstetric Levator Ani Muscle Injuries: Current Status," *Ultrasound Obstetrics and Gynecology* 39 (2012): 372–383.

11. A Vleeming et al., "European Guidelines for the Diagnosis and Treatment of Pelvic Girdle Pain," *European Spine Journal* 17 (2008): 794–819.

12. EA McDonald et al., "Dyspareunia and Childbirth: A Prospective Cohort Study," *British Journal of Obstetrics and Gynecology* 21 January 2015, doi: 10.1111/1471-0528.13263.

2

HOW DID I GET PELVIC PAIN? THE IMPORTANCE OF UNCOVERING CONTRIBUTING FACTORS

HOW DID I GET PELVIC PAIN?

This is a question that every person dealing with pelvic pain asks, and more so than the question *"What is my diagnosis?"* it's important to answer, because the information plays a key role in treatment. In general, the reality is that for most people with pelvic pain, it's not just one thing that caused their pelvic pain, but a handful of underlying causes that collectively provoked their symptoms. Remember, pelvic pain is often a muscle-driven pain syndrome, so when we talk about "contributing factors," what we're really talking about are the various events—childbirth, surgery, a fall on the tailbone, an infection, even repetitive activities like bicycling or sitting for long periods of time—that can cause the pelvic floor to become impaired. So *contributing factors* are what ultimately cause the *pelvic floor neuromuscular impairments* that in turn cause *the symptoms* of pelvic pain. Take Paul for example. Paul is a high-powered attorney in his forties whose job requires countless hours of sitting at a desk, in courtrooms, and on airplanes. Over the years, the contributing factor of sitting for long periods of time caused Paul's pelvic floor muscles to become overly tight. These too-tight muscles served as the impairment, which led to the development of his pelvic pain symptoms—anal and sit bone pain.

In this chapter, we're shining the spotlight on contributing factors. As mentioned above, it's an important variable of the pelvic pain equation to understand, because identifying all the factors that contribute to a patient's pelvic pain is a vital part of the treatment process. If the contributing factors, aka the underlying causes, of a patient's pelvic pain are not addressed, then the patient has less of a chance of getting better and/or more of a chance of recurring symptoms. Another reason it's important for patients to understand all the factors contributing to their symptoms is that it gives them the information they need to best advocate for their recovery. We'll start off the chapter with a basic explanation of how a contributing factor, whether it's a series of infections or a hormonal imbalance, actually evolves into a symptom-causing impairment. From there we'll take a look at the slew of contributing factors that can play a role in pelvic pain. What's so striking about this list is its variability; while some of the items on the list may seem obvious, others will come as a complete surprise to many readers. Lastly, we'll explore how, more often than not, it's a "perfect storm" of contributing factors that kicks off a pelvic pain syndrome.

HOW A CONTRIBUTING FACTOR BECOMES AN IMPAIRMENT

The straining that accompanies chronic constipation, the searing pain brought on by repetitive urinary tract infections (UTIs), the pushing that occurs with childbirth, the tissue compression that occurs with long hours of sitting; how can these events turn into the neuromuscular impairments that cause the symptoms of pelvic pain? While there are a few different ways, in this section we're going to focus on two of the most common ways. The first has to do with the way muscles work and the second has to do with the intimate relationship between organs and the tissue that surrounds them. Let's start with the former. Muscles are made up of fibers that either overlap to contract (shorten) the muscle or pull apart to stretch (lengthen) the muscle. Muscles that become too short because the fibers begin to overlap too much (as can occur with clenching) or too long because the fibers pull too far apart (as can occur with pushing during childbirth or constipation) become vulnerable to the development of trigger points. (As mentioned in a previous chapter, trigger points, a common impairment contributing to pelvic pain, are small, taut patches of painful, involuntarily contracted muscle fibers.) On top of the development of painful trigger points, muscles that become too short in and of themselves cause pelvic pain primarily because they restrict blood flow to the area.

The second main way a contributing factor becomes an impairment involves the intimate relationship between internal organs and the soft tissue surrounding them. As we discussed in chapter 1, the pelvic floor encapsulates a host of different organs, such as the uterus in women, the prostate in men, and the bladder and bowels in both men and women. When a problem arises with any of these organs, such as when the bladder and urethra are inflamed due to a UTI, pain from the organs can be referred to the surrounding neuromuscular tissue, namely the pelvic floor muscles and nerves, the abdominal muscles, and even the skin, such as the skin of the vulva or the penis. More familiar examples of organ-tissue referral patterns are when a person has a heart attack and pain is felt in the neck, shoulders, and/or back rather than the chest. Why does this pain referral happen? Researchers are not entirely sure, but an overriding theory is that at the level of the spinal cord there is crosstalk between the organs that are in trouble and the soft tissue and nerves located near them. Basically, the pain signal originating from the organ becomes jumbled, causing pain to be felt in areas other than where it stems. In addition to pain referral from organs, this crisscrossing of spinal cord signals can actually cause the pelvic floor muscles to contract. As a result, repetitive UTIs, for example, can cause the pelvic floor tissue and muscles to become too tight. On the flip side, impaired tissue of the pelvic floor can have this same reflexive effect on nearby organs. For example, tight pelvic floor muscles can cause pain in the urethra, bladder, or rectum. This in turn can create symptoms that mimic a urinary tract infection or gastrointestinal distress. None of these mechanisms are the patients' fault. We point this out because often we have patients who blame themselves for "clenching" in response to events, like a series of infections or endometriosis, wrongly believing that if only they'd been more "relaxed" and "less anxious" during these events, they wouldn't have gotten pelvic pain. This is simply not the case. These are physiological responses, which we have no conscious control over.

CONTRIBUTING FACTORS

Now that we've discussed how a contributing factor becomes an impairment, let's take a look at the varied list of factors that can contribute to pelvic pain. As we already touched on in the last chapter, the pelvic floor is a major hub of the body. Not only does it play a major role in daily movement, like walking and running, sitting, and standing, it also plays a starring role in many important bodily functions, including sexual activity, bowel movements, and urination. Is it any wonder then that so many different events can contribute to a pelvic pain syndrome? The list below covers the most common factors in pelvic pain, and while some of the items on it, like prolonged pushing during childbirth, might seem obvious, others, like having one leg that's shorter than the other, training for a marathon, or going through menopause, will likely come as a surprise to many readers.

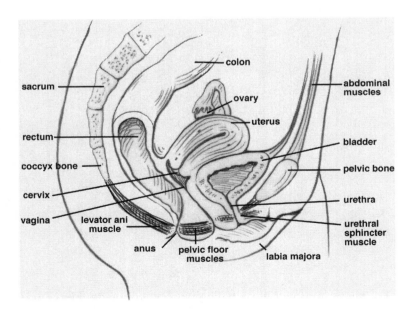

Figure 2.1.   Urogynecological midsaggital view of the female pelvis. *Source: Amy Stein, DPT, BCB-PMD*

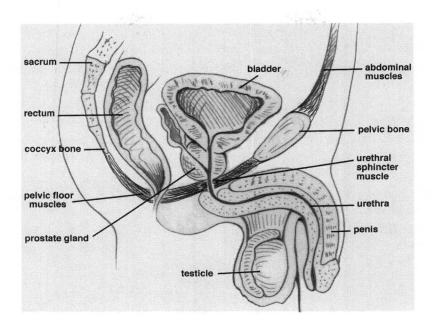

Figure 2.2. Urogenital midsaggital view of the male pelvis. *Source: Amy Stein, DPT, BCB-PMD*

Infections

A handful of different infections can contribute to pelvic pain. These include urinary tract infections (UTIs) and vaginal infections, such as those caused by yeast or bacteria. In addition, infectious agents can attack glands in the area, such as the prostate gland in men and the Bartholin's glands in women. (The Bartholin's glands are two pea-size glands located on either side of the opening of the vagina that secrete fluid to help lubricate the vagina for sex. These glands can become blocked and develop cysts, which can in turn become inflamed and infected.) Any of these infections can kick off any one or a combination of the mechanisms explained above, which then can lead to the neuromuscular impairments that cause pelvic pain. For example, a woman gets a UTI, which causes her bladder and urethra to become inflamed, causing urethral burning as well as pain in her lower abdomen. As a result, the connective tissue around her urethra as well as the muscles in her lower abdomen and groin become restricted, causing an additional source of pain. A UTI can also have symptoms of urinary urgency and frequency, which can cause a "holding" or clench response with the same outcome: muscles that become too tight, lack of blood flow, and vulnerability to trigger points. Another example is a man who gets chlamydia, a common sexually transmitted disease, and clenches his pelvic floor muscles because of the inflammation and pain from the infection. (This clenching is referred to as "guarding." Guarding is when we unconsciously clench our muscles to protect an area of the body that is inflamed or injured. Although it starts off as a protective mechanism, guarding ultimately causes muscles to become too tight—remember those overlapping muscle fibers—setting the stage for pain.)

Another way an infection can play a role in pelvic pain is when a woman gets multiple yeast infections. Here's how: over time, multiple yeast infections can cause neural irritation, either in major nerve branches of the pelvic floor, such as the pudendal nerve, or within the smaller, more superficial nerves that feed the skin of the vulva. This nerve irritation can cause pain in any of the areas these nerves innervate, such as the skin of the vulva, the skin of the clitoris, the perineum, the vagina, the urethra, and/or the rectum, as well as the guarding pattern described above.

In all the scenarios described above, even after the infection itself has cleared up, the resulting neuromuscular impairments can stick around, even mimicking the symptoms of the infection. While it's possible for one relatively normal infection to cause this outcome, more often than not, a severe infection that lasts a long time or a series of infections suffered over a period of years are the culprits. If it is determined that an infection is an underlying cause of a patient's pelvic pain, it's important that the infection be successfully treated by a doctor in order for recovery to occur. And if a patient is getting recurrent infections, such as recurrent UTIs after sex, it's important to work with a physician to figure out why this is happening and to take preventive measures.

Surgery

Dozens of different surgeries impact the pelvic floor. Some of the more common ones are hysterectomy, surgery to correct pelvic organ prolapse, hernia repair, and prostatectomy. So how can a surgery contribute to pelvic pain? The basic explanation is that an event can occur as a result of either the specific surgery itself (for example, the mesh used in a surgery to correct a pelvic organ prolapse can entrap a nerve) or the positioning of the patient during the surgery (such as the specific position of the hip joint during a hip labral repair). More often than not, when a surgery is behind pelvic pain symptoms, the patient will notice symptoms immediately after the surgical procedure. But sometimes there is a time lag. For instance, with mesh placement to correct a pelvic organ prolapse, problems might not arise until scarring starts to form around the mesh. Whatever the specifics of the case, if a patient believes that unresolved pelvic pain following surgery was caused by the surgery, we recommend that he/she consult with their physician as well as seek a second opinion. In these situations, it is possible that a follow-up surgery can decrease or eliminate the patient's pelvic pain, such as removal of mesh placement; therefore, it may be useful to consult a pelvic pain surgical specialist in this case.

Scar Tissue

Scar tissue is a common contributing factor to pelvic pain. Scar tissue is fibrous tissue that replaces normal tissue after an injury. It's made of the same stuff as the tissue it replaces—collagen. However, the quality of the collagen is inferior to the tissue it replaces. Plus, the tissue is usually not as elastic as the original. Scarring that affects the pelvic floor can happen as a result of any trauma to the area, including a C-section, perineum tear, or episiotomy during childbirth as well as a prostatectomy, a hysterectomy, a vasectomy, bowel surgery, endometriosis surgery, or a Bartholin's gland abscess removal. Scarring can also result from a skin disease called lichen sclerosis that can affect the vulva.

There are three major ways that scarring within or adjacent to the pelvic floor can cause problems. First, scar tissue is indiscriminate in what it attaches to. So it can adhere to skin, muscle, or connective tissue. Wherever it decides to hang out, it pulls on the surrounding tissue, making the area taut and restricting blood flow, which often results in pain. Another way that scar tissue can wreak havoc within the pelvic floor is as a result of referred pain. Remember, a network of nerves innervates the pelvic floor. If a scar is on top of or impinging on a nerve that innervates another part of the pelvic floor, then that area can also be affected. For example, if a man has a surgery to repair an inguinal hernia (a condition in which soft tissue bulges through the lower abdominal wall or groin), the mesh used in the surgery could entrap the ilioinguinal nerve located in the wall of the abdomen, causing pain in the root of the penis or the upper part of the scrotum. That's why it's important to remember that the pain and dysfunction caused by a scar is not always going to be in the area where the scar is. Another way scar tissue can cause problems within the pelvic floor is by impairing function in the area where it's located. For instance, if a muscle is torn and then a scar forms, as in an anal sphincter tear during a difficult childbirth, that muscle may lose some of its ability to contract, which can lead to a loss of control over urination, bowel movements, or sexual function.

Pregnancy/Childbirth

When a woman goes through a pregnancy and delivers a baby, her pelvic floor is put through the wringer. This is why we've decided to devote an entire chapter (chapter 4) to the topic of pregnancy and the pelvic floor. Common pelvic pain–related symptoms women can experience as a result of pregnancy and childbirth include back, groin, hip, vulvovaginal, tailbone, or pelvic floor pain; pain during sex; diminished or absent orgasm; urinary frequency, urgency, or retention (retention is difficulty starting the urine stream); constipation; and difficulty evacuating stool. Plus, vaginal tearing or an episiotomy during a vaginal delivery can also cause future issues with pelvic floor muscles.

Constipation

Constipation plays a major role in pelvic pain. But unlike some of the other contributing factors described in this chapter, it can either contribute to pelvic pain *or* be a symptom of other neuromuscular impairments. There are two different types of constipation. The first is general constipation, caused by a lack of motility in the large intestine. The large intestine, aka the colon, is designed to carry out a contracting and squeezing motion that propels stool through it. This action can become impaired, causing stool to move excessively slowly or not much at all. A variety of things can lead to this type of constipation, such as poor diet, lack of fluid intake, lack of exercise, or a sluggish colon. Also, many kinds of medication, like opiates or other pain meds, can cause general constipation. The second type of constipation is known as outlet constipation. Outlet constipation occurs when stool sits in the rectum and is difficult to eliminate. In other words, the train makes it to the station, but then gets stuck there. This can be due to pelvic floor muscle dysfunction, an overstretched rectum, or a situation in women where the tissue that separates the vaginal and rectal canals becomes weak. When stool becomes stuck, we tend to want to bear down and push in an effort to pass it. But straining only makes matters worse; the more we push, the more muscles and tissue become strained in both men and women. And in women, over time, the tissue between the vagina and rectum can even weaken, further exacerbating constipation. In this case, not only is stool having a hard time getting through the external sphincter, it's getting stuck and pocketing in weakened tissue.

Vulvovaginal/Anal Fissures

A vulvovaginal fissure is a tear or crack in the lining of the vulvovaginal tissue, while an anal fissure is a tear in the lining of the anal canal. Some of the more common reasons for vulvovaginal fissures are a lack of tissue integrity due to a drop in estrogen levels, frequent yeast infections, or decreased lubrication. As for anal fissures, more often than not, repetitive straining because of chronic constipation is the culprit. Fissures themselves can be very painful, causing sharp, stinging, burning pain as well as itching and bleeding. But as with any other contributing factor, they can also cause secondary pain due to their impact on the pelvic floor muscles. For instance, the pain from the fissure will cause guarding, which in turn will cause all the issues that come along with too-tight pelvic floor muscles. If vulvovaginal fissures are an underlying factor in a woman's pain, she should seek help from either a gynecologist or a dermatologist specializing in vulvovaginal skin issues (while these specialists are rare, they do exist). Anal fissures are treated by a colorectal doctor.

Anatomical/Biomechanical Abnormalities

A slew of anatomical/biomechanical abnormalities, such as having one leg that's shorter than the other, contribute to pelvic pain. (An anatomical abnormality is a problem with how the body is structured, whereas a biomechanical abnormality is a problem that affects how the body moves.) So why do anatomical/biomechanical abnormalities so often play a role in pelvic pain? The reason has to do with how the pelvic girdle (the "pelvic girdle" is all the pelvic floor muscles, the muscles that attach to the pelvis, and the basin-shaped unit of bones between the trunk and the legs) interacts with the rest of the body. The muscles of the pelvic girdle are always activated, whether it's to make sure we remain continent or to give us stability for standing up or walking. Therefore, a problem with another part of the body, such as when a person has poor posture, can actually affect the pelvic girdle. Whether or not it will ultimately contribute to pelvic pain depends on the severity and duration of the issue as well as the person's behavior. Some common anatomical/biomechanical abnormalities include sacroiliac joint dysfunction, spine dysfunction and/or pathology, postural dysfunction, limited or excessive joint mobility, and scoliosis (curvature of the spine). Plus, any orthopedic issue, such as a knee issue, also fits into this category. That's because a hip, knee, or back injury can change a person's anatomical structure in a way that can contribute to pelvic pain. One example is piriformis syndrome, which occurs when the sciatic nerve (a long nerve that begins in the low back and runs through the buttocks and all the way down to the lower limbs) is compressed or irritated by the piriformis muscle and other muscles that surround it in the buttocks. Because it's located in the vicinity of this problem, the obturator internus muscle (a thick, fan-shaped muscle within the pelvic floor) in someone with piriformis syndrome may become too tight, causing pelvic pain symptoms, such as tailbone or anal pain, or pain with sitting. Sometimes a patient has had a lifelong issue that suddenly becomes a problem. Oftentimes a patient will make the point that they've had the issue their whole life, so why is it a problem now? Our response is, "While it's existed for your whole life, in the past it hasn't caused you any problems. Now it's contributing to your pelvic pain, and in order to get you better, we have to work to normalize this anatomic issue." An anatomic deviation can become an issue over time or be provoked by something such as more time sitting or even getting a new car with a different type of seat. In addition, anatomical/biomechanical abnormalities can by themselves cause pelvic pain, or they can predispose someone to pelvic pain, if and when other factors come into play.

For example, let's say a woman has hypermobile joints, meaning her ligaments are too loose, and her muscles have to work harder to keep the joint the muscles surround together and functional. This woman gets a series of yeast infections, which make her pelvic floor muscles even tighter. Because of the hypermobility she has had her whole life, her pelvic floor muscles are already on the tight side, making her more likely to get pain from tight muscles than a woman who had the same series of infections but didn't already have tight muscles. So the series of yeast infections compound an already bad situation, causing an onset of pain. To treat this patient's pelvic pain, we'll have to work on the muscle dysfunction her hypermobility has caused over her entire life.

Overuse Injury

If a person is predisposed to pelvic pain due to an anatomical/biomechanical abnormality or any other issue, such as overly tight muscles from repetitive yeast infections, overuse injuries can occur, which in turn can contribute to the development of pelvic pain. The term "overuse" refers to any activity that exceeds a particular muscle's capabilities. For example, if someone has tight pelvic floor muscles, for whatever reason, and begins to do a popular high-intensity workout called Cross-Fit training, he/she might be susceptible to developing pelvic pain, whereas a person with a perfectly normal pelvic floor will have no problem with the workout. To be sure, often changes to a person's daily routine, which result in an overuse injury, act as the catalyst for pelvic pain. These changes can include taking up cycling, Pilates, or yoga; driving a new car; starting a long commute to work; or weathering a bad cough. But of course it doesn't have to be a new activity. It could be an activity a person has been doing for years, like a golfer who's had the same swing for years, a skateboarder who always pushes off with the same leg, or horseback riding or cycling that eventually catches up with his/her pelvic floor.

Hormonal Issues (in Women)

Because of their adjacency to the pelvic floor nerves and muscles, the vulvar and vaginal tissue, if compromised, can play a role in pelvic pain. And one of the things that can compromise vulvar/vaginal tissue is hormone fluctuation, specifically a drop in estrogen. For example, a drop in estrogen, as can occur either during perimenopause or menopause, can cause vulvar/vaginal tissue to have less skin integrity, which can result in skin tears (fissures) and/or pain with intercourse. As a result, pelvic floor muscle guarding can occur, setting the woman up for pelvic pain. In addition, an estrogen drop decreases a woman's ability to naturally lubricate, also causing pain with intercourse. Besides perimenopause and menopause, other hormonal issues that can contribute to pelvic pain include thyroid disease, starting a new birth control pill, and taking birth control for an extended period of time. For its part, thyroid disease is associated with all muscle pain, pelvic pain included. As for birth control pills and pelvic pain, generally, they can affect hormone levels, but to what extent they do so is very individual. However, we'd like to mention another issue surrounding birth control pills and pelvic pain. It involves an ongoing controversy in the pelvic pain arena. Here's the lowdown: aside from their obvious role in preventing unwanted pregnancy, birth control pills are the first-line treatment for several painful gynecologic diseases, such as endometriosis. This is because they suppress the hormones that perpetuate these diseases. However, this hormone suppression doesn't just have an effect on the reproductive tract; it also affects the tissue, muscle, or glands under its influence. Emerging research suggests that birth control pills can have a negative impact on vulvar and periurethral tissues and other glands in the pelvic region, and that this may actually cause pelvic pain. According to the theory, certain women may be more genetically susceptible to developing pelvic pain from oral contraceptives than others.[1] When it comes to the birth control pill as it may or may not relate to pelvic pain, our advice is if a woman develops pelvic pain after starting or stopping the birth control pill, hormonal deficiencies from the pill may be a factor in her pain, and she should definitely talk to her gynecologist about it. Or if she suspects that long-term birth control use may be contributing to her pain, she should also consult her gynecologist. And overall, if a hormonal issue is contributing to a patient's pain, it's important for her to see a physician, typically either a gynecologist or an endocrinologist, to get the problem under control.

Diseases/Syndromes

A handful of diseases/syndromes can have an impact on the pelvic floor, acting as contributing factors to pelvic pain. The most common of these are endometriosis, irritable bowel syndrome, fibromyalgia, polycystic ovarian syndrome, and interstitial cystitis. These conditions tend to cause symptoms that in turn create pain-causing impairments to the pelvic floor. For an example, let's look at how endometriosis can contribute to pelvic pain. Endometriosis is a condition where tissue like that which lines the inside of the uterus (known as endometrial tissue) grows outside of the uterus, most commonly in the abdominal cavity. This tissue can implant on any surface within the abdominal cavity, including the ovaries, bladder, rectum, and the abdominal/pelvic wall. Commonly reported symptoms of endometriosis are painful cramping prior to menstruation, pain during menstruation, pain with sex, bladder pain, and painful bowel movements. Endometriosis can impact the pelvic floor and cause pain in a variety of ways. First, endometrial tissue bleeds with menstruation, often leading to inflammation, scar tissue, and adhesion formation inside the abdominal and pelvic cavities. (Adhesions are fibrous bands of scar tissue that can attach to organs, muscles, and fascia.) These areas can become a source of pain. Furthermore, this can set up an unhealthy environment within the pelvic floor and pelvic girdle muscles because the decrease in pelvic and abdominal organ/muscle/connective tissue mobility can lead to decreased circulation, too-tight muscles, the development of painful trigger points, and connective tissue restriction. So on top of all the symptoms that already come with endometriosis, a patient can develop a host of pelvic floor–related impairments that cause pain on top of an already painful situation. In addition to the specific ways a particular disease process can contribute to pelvic pain, such as mentioned above in the case of endometriosis, in general, any painful symptoms that come along with a condition can lead to involuntary muscle contraction and guarding behaviors, further exacerbating the situation.

THE PERFECT STORM

As you can see after reading this chapter, a host of different factors can contribute to a pelvic pain syndrome. It's important for both providers and patients to have them on their radar in order to have all the information necessary to put together the best treatment plan. Equally important is fully understanding *how* a pelvic pain syndrome typically occurs. More often than not, it's not just one of the contributing factors discussed above that causes a full-blown pelvic pain syndrome; it's a handful of factors coupled with a timing component. Indeed, oftentimes several things have to happen at an exact moment in time for a person to develop pelvic pain. We call this a "perfect storm" scenario. Here's an example. Kathy, a 19-year-old college sophomore, gets mononucleosis, aka "mono." As a result of the virus, she develops a persistent cervical infection, which is treated with several rounds of antibiotics. Due to the antibiotics she gets thrush (a yeast infection in the mouth) as well as a vaginal yeast infection. Many rounds of antifungals later to treat what becomes a chronic vaginal yeast infection, she begins to have pain with intercourse. The pain with intercourse, along with the chronic yeast infections, causes Kathy to clench her pelvic floor muscles. On top of all that, Kathy is very hypermobile. So add tight pelvic floor muscles to pelvic girdle muscles that are already overworking to keep pelvic joints together, and what you get is even more pelvic floor muscle dysfunction. So what you end up with is a series of events—a virus that caused a yeast infection that kicked off muscle clenching that, when combined with an anatomical abnormality, caused muscle tightness—which ultimately created the perfect storm that left symptoms of pelvic pain in its wake.

TONY'S STORY

I've always been a super-athletic guy. When I wasn't chasing after my kids or helping to run my family's business, you could find me surfing, hunting, snowboarding, golfing, swimming, or playing basketball. But my active lifestyle came to a screeching halt when I was 29, and there was a period of time when I was sure I'd never participate in another activity I loved again, let alone be able to work or even have relations with my wife. It all started one unseasonably warm afternoon in February. On that day, as usual, I was in active mode, attempting to pull off the perfect handstand, when all of a sudden, I felt a sharp pinching pain in my lower abs. Three doctors later, I was diagnosed with an "abdominal strain" and prescribed core-strengthening exercises. The exercises only made my pain worse, and in a matter of weeks my symptoms exploded. The pain in my lower abdomen snowballed into pain with sitting, constant perineum and groin pain, and a burning pain at the tip of my penis as well as occasional anal pain. Unable to find any answers from the doctors I visited, I turned to the Internet. That's when the fear and panic set in. After spending hours online, I discovered that my symptoms were a match with a disorder called "pudendal nerve entrapment" or "PNE." After reading a litany of stories about PNE, I became convinced that I needed surgery as soon as possible to free an entrapped pudendal nerve. Otherwise, according to the information I was reading online, my symptoms would continue to get worse. I even contacted one of the doctors mentioned in the online forums who performed the surgery. The doctor encouraged me to fly out and schedule the surgery with him right away. I was terrified. I was reading all these horror stories, and I believed that if I didn't get surgery as soon as possible, I would end up impotent and incontinent. Even with surgery I was afraid of what my life was going to become. However, before I signed up for surgery, I decided to see one more doctor in San Francisco. Thankfully, that doctor was in the know about male pelvic pain. The doctor explained that trigger points and tight muscles in the pelvic floor and/or abdomen have the potential to cause all the symptoms I was experiencing. The doctor then prescribed pelvic floor PT. I admit at first I didn't believe PT was going to help me. But I decided I'd give it a try as a final effort before I got the surgery. After my first session with Stephanie, I felt a slight bit of relief, which was encouraging. What Stephanie found were trigger points throughout my rectus abdominus muscle, likely caused by the 200 crunches I did about four to five times a week. In addition, she found a great deal of external connective tissue restriction and pelvic floor muscle tightness as well as some irritation of my pudendal nerve. She also uncovered clues that my issues had been bubbling for some time before finally coming up to the surface. For one thing, I had a history of constipation and low back pain. For another thing, the urinary frequency I'd experience after long bike rides and the occasional post-ejaculatory burning I felt were signs that I had had underlying pelvic floor impairments for years. Ultimately, with regular PT sessions—at first twice weekly and then weekly—my pain and symptoms began to diminish, until eventually they were gone altogether. Today I have zero pain and I'm living an unrestricted, active life. But it didn't go away overnight. It took time, patience, and a lot of commitment to treatment.

CONCLUSION

Uncovering a patient's contributing factors and putting together the history of his/her "perfect storm" is one of the most important prerequisites of putting a treatment plan into action. It's a process that the patient and his/her PT, and other providers, must commit to together. Our hope is that this chapter will help with that process. In addition to our exploration of all the factors that can contribute to pelvic pain, we touched on the neuromuscular impairments that so often are in the driver's seat of a patient's pain. In the next chapter, we're going to take a closer look at those neuromuscular impairments by explaining exactly what can go wrong with the pelvic floor muscles, nerves, and connective tissue to cause the variety of symptoms that can make up a pelvic pain syndrome.

3

DEMYSTIFYING THE NEUROMUSCULAR IMPAIRMENTS THAT CAUSE PELVIC PAIN

When someone has back pain, knee pain, or shoulder pain, their mind immediately goes to the neuromuscular system. *Is it a muscular issue? A problem with the nerves of the area? Are joints or ligaments involved?* But when symptoms of pelvic pain arise—vaginal burning, anal pain, post-ejaculatory burning, testicular pain, pain with urination—the first stop on the thought train is rarely the neuromuscular system. And for many it can take a pretty long time to get there, with frustrating detours along the way. Even when it *is* put on the table as the possible driver of pain, some patients still have a hard time wrapping their heads around it. Take Mary for instance, a patient in her thirties who suffered from vulvar and urethral burning as well as urinary urgency/frequency. The first doctor Mary saw actually did tell her that he believed her muscles were tight and gave her a referral to a pelvic floor PT. However, she visited two more doctors and the emergency room before she finally decided to give the PT a call, and not because she really believed it was her answer. It was more a matter of needing to do something and figuring she might as well try a different route than the one she had already taken. When asked why she hesitated to see the PT, she simply said, "I just couldn't understand how PT, where you go when you need your knee or shoulder or leg fixed, was going to help with my burning vulva and urethra!" This is a completely understandable sentiment. The reality is that we simply aren't used to associating most of the areas of the body impacted by pelvic pain with muscles, nerves, and connective tissue. It just doesn't compute. This is why we've decided to devote an entire chapter to a discussion of how neuromuscular impairments can and do drive pelvic pain. In the previous chapter we talked about how different events can cause the neuromuscular impairments that in turn cause the symptoms of pelvic pain. In this chapter, we're drilling down a little deeper to take a look at exactly how these neuromuscular impairments translate into pelvic pain. Gaining this level of understanding is important, not only for the reasons we mention above, but also because it removes the mystery and sinisterness that so often surrounds persistent pelvic pain. For instance, when Mary learned that trigger points and too-tight muscles were the main drivers of her pain, she said it was a huge relief. "I wasn't crazy!" she said. "There wasn't some mysterious force causing my pain. There were actual physiological impairments at play, and they were treatable."

We'll begin the chapter with a discussion of what can go wrong with the muscles of the pelvic floor to cause pelvic pain. Next, we'll tackle the nerve issues that can come into play. From there we'll take a look at how connective tissue causes symptoms. Lastly, we'll end the chapter with an explanation of how the central nervous system enters into the mix. This chapter lays the groundwork for chapters 7 and 8, which go into detail on how all these impairments are treated.

MUSCLE IMPAIRMENTS

Too-Tight Muscles

As we've already explained, the hammock-like bundle of muscles that make up the pelvic floor support organs, assist in urinary and fecal continence, aid in sexual functioning, and stabilize connecting joints. And these muscles are always active, because if they were to completely relax, incontinence and organ prolapse would ensue. This constant state of contraction is actually what makes them more challenging to treat when they become impaired. As we've already touched on in previous chapters, two main impairments impact the muscles of the pelvic floor: too-tight muscles and trigger points.

Let's talk too-tight muscles first. In the last chapter we talked about what causes pelvic floor muscles to become too tight, but so far we haven't really delved into exactly why those tight muscles cause pain. The overriding reason is that when muscles become too tight, blood flow becomes restricted, meaning less oxygen reaches the tissue. This oxygen deficiency causes pain. In addition, too-tight muscles can actually cause other impairments that also cause pain. So you end up with pain on top of pain. For instance, tight muscles have a tendency to develop trigger points, a situation that also causes pain as well as dysfunction such as urinary urgency/frequency. This situation can also cause the compression of surrounding nerves, again, causing pain. On top of all that, tight muscles don't function efficiently, putting them at greater risk of incurring damage, like strains or tears, both of which, you guessed it, cause pain and dysfunction.

And tight muscles don't just cause pain where they lie; they also affect surrounding tissue. In the last chapter, we talked about how tight muscles can cause pain/dysfunction in adjacent organs, like when the muscles around the urinary sphincter become too tight, causing urgency, frequency, or pain with urination, but in addition to that, tight muscles can put the muscles they work closely with at risk. For example, neighboring muscles are going to have to compensate for a tight muscle that isn't "pulling its weight," so to speak. This in turn can cause pain in these muscles. To add insult to injury, too-tight pelvic floor muscles can also become weak muscles, meaning they aren't able to contract adequately. A consequence of this could be incontinence. Many pelvic pain symptoms are caused by too-tight muscles, including:

- Difficulty starting urine stream and interrupted urine stream
- Post-void "dribble"
- "Pinching" in the urethra after voiding
- Vulvar pain or burning
- Vulvar pain and/or deep vaginal pain with intercourse
- Perineal pain
- Pain at sit bones or tailbone when sitting
- Diminished or painful orgasm
- Trouble evacuating stool

WHY KEGELS ARE BAD FOR YOUR TIGHT PELVIC FLOOR

For decades doctors, PTs, trainers, therapists, you name it, have been hammering away at women—and men too—to do their Kegels to strengthen their pelvic floors. Preventing incontinence after childbirth and better sex are the promise for taking this advice. To be sure, it's advice that's seeped into mainstream culture. But the fact of the matter is Kegels are NOT for everybody, and for a certain population, doing them will actually do harm, not good. People with too-tight pelvic floor muscles and/or trigger points in their pelvic floor muscles should not do Kegels. Here's why: when you do a Kegel, you're doing a muscle contraction, and if you already have a tight pelvic floor, contracting it will only make it tighter, making your pelvic floor problems worse. Tight muscles do not like to be squeezed further. Not to mention that if you are predisposed to pelvic pain, perhaps your pelvic floor is tight but not yet symptomatic. Kegels could push you to develop symptoms. Remember, your pelvic floor muscles are the only group of muscles in the body that never get to rest, ever. They're working all the time to maintain continence, to support our pelvic organs, and to contribute to our posture and stability. Therefore, these muscles are "working out" all the time and don't follow the same rules as the other muscle groups in the body. Therefore, if you do get carried away with Kegels and over-strengthen your pelvic floor muscles, they can become too tight, which in turn can cause dysfunction and symptoms, such as pain and urinary urgency and frequency. So the pelvic floor muscles do not need extra strengthening from doing Kegels, unless something has overstretched them or injured them in some way that has made them truly weak (not weak *and tight*, but more on that in a bit). Your pelvic floor muscles can become overstretched and/or weak after childbirth, with age-related changes that are exacerbated by the hormonal changes during menopause, and after some gynecological surgeries. And this overstretching and weakening can lead to incontinence and pelvic organ prolapse. Kegels are appropriate when the pelvic floor is truly weak and/or overstretched. We prescribe them all the time for this patient demographic. So tight muscles = Kegels bad. Weak and/or overstretched muscles = Kegels okay. If only we could end things here. But by now you're probably on to the fact that things are seldom simple with the pelvic floor. So here's the clincher: it's possible for a weak pelvic floor to also be a tight pelvic floor and/or to contain trigger points. In this situation, it's definitely NOT okay to do Kegels. So what does someone who has both a tight and a weak pelvic floor do, especially if he/she has other symptoms caused by the weakness? Well, the appropriate course of action in this situation would be to first work to clear up the tightness and trigger points with PT and whatever other treatments are appropriate. And then once the pelvic floor muscles are at a healthy tone—no longer too tight/all trigger points are gone—do Kegel exercises recommended by a trained PT to strengthen your pelvic floor. So to summarize: Kegels are not appropriate for folks with a tight pelvic floor or active trigger points or folks with a weak AND a tight pelvic floor. But it's okay to do Kegels to strengthen a weak pelvic floor.

TRIGGER POINTS

Before we talk about what causes trigger points or the role they play in pelvic pain, let's first take a closer look at what a trigger point is. As we've already mentioned, a trigger point is a small, taut band of involuntarily contracted muscle fibers within a muscle. But why do these contracted muscle fibers cause pain? The reason is that they affect blood supply to the nearby tissue (sound familiar?), which in turn makes the area hyperirritable, which will become even more uncomfortable/painful if compressed. They also cause referred pain to other areas. Two leading medical professionals, Drs. David Simons and Janet Travell, first coined the term "trigger point" in 1942. What they found in their research was that a handful of different kinds of trigger points exist. For instance, there are active trigger points, which as their name suggests, actively cause pain and other symptoms; latent trigger points, which are dormant but have the potential to cause trouble if they become activated; and satellite trigger points, which can crop up in another trigger point's referral zone.[1] (More on trigger point referral zones in a bit.) As we've already mentioned, muscles that are too tight, overlengthened, or weak are vulnerable to developing trigger points. Repetitive motions can lead to muscles that are too tight or overlengthened. For example, repetitively straining to have a bowel movement can lead to an overlengthening of the pelvic floor muscles. Also, when a checkout clerk regularly rotates to one side to scan items, muscles can become too tight on the side contracting to cause the rotation. In both scenarios the pelvic floor muscles are now vulnerable to developing trigger points because their ability to function properly becomes compromised and they become strained. In addition to repetitive behaviors/ movements, trigger points can crop up for other reasons. For example, local trauma can injure healthy muscles, causing trigger points to form. Examples of such trauma include a fall on the tailbone or childbirth. If muscles are already vulnerable due to an overshortening or overlengthening issue, seemingly benign things like a colonoscopy, laparoscopic surgery, or vaginal ultrasound can cause a trigger point. Plus, mechanical or organic stressors, like a hip labral tear or endometriosis, can also cause the development of trigger points.

Trigger points can be very misleading, and when dealing with them, it's a mistake to always assume the problem is where the pain is. For instance, they often refer pain elsewhere. For example, trigger points in the obturator internus muscle of the pelvic floor (a primary hip muscle that rotates the hip outward) can refer pain to the tailbone or the area above the opening of the anus. In addition to pain referral to these areas, a trigger point in the obturator internus muscle can cause pudendal nerve irritation because of its proximity to the pudendal nerve. On top of all that, trigger points can mimic joint pain and contribute to joint dysfunction because they cause altered movement patterns. For example, let's say you have trigger points in your gluteal muscles, specifically your gluteus maximus muscles, whose job it is to extend your hips. Because they have trigger points in them, these muscles are unable to function normally. Specifically, they are unable to recruit or activate normally when they need to during walking, causing your body to make adjustments. Indeed, in order to walk you have to be able to extend your hip to propel yourself forward. If your gluteus maximus isn't working correctly to do that, other muscles (for example, your iliotibial band, commonly referred to as the "IT band," which is a long, very tough muscle along the side of your leg that runs from your hip to your knee) are going to help out. Say this has been going on for months, or even years. The IT band will get tighter and tighter over time. Eventually it will start pulling on the kneecap, which can ultimately lead to knee pain. Trigger points can also refer pain to nearby organ systems and create connective tissue restrictions in overlying connective tissue.

Pretty much everyone will deal with trigger points at some point in their lives. The good news is that even though some 620 potential trigger points are possible in human muscle, they show up in pretty much the same location in everyone based on where nerves enter the muscles. Where they refer pain is also based on neurologic connections; therefore, trigger point maps exist, complete with referral patterns, and that goes for the pelvic floor too. This is great news, because as PTs undergo training to identify trigger points, they learn common trigger point locations that are associated with particular symptoms. This allows them to initiate a treatment plan that will likely start providing relief sooner rather than later. Trigger points play a role in the vast majority of cases of pelvic pain. Indeed, in some cases, they're the only culprits. For instance, we had a male patient, Ben, who had trigger points in his rectus abdominis muscle (the "six-pack" muscles of the abdomen) from doing too many sit-ups over a period of years. His main complaints were lower abdominal pain and penile pain. Initially he was misdiagnosed

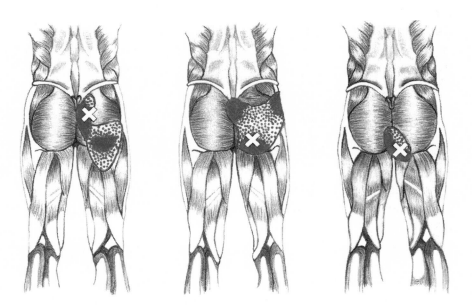

Figure 3.1. Gluteus maximus muscle trigger points and their referral pattern. "X" indicates the trigger point, the solid shaded area indicates the primary referral zone, and the dotted area indicates the secondary referral zone. *Source: Pelvic Health and Rehabilitation Center*

with a hernia. He found his way to our clinic, and after about three months of working to release those trigger points, Ben's symptoms resolved. However, while it's possible for trigger points to be the sole cause of someone's pelvic pain, it's much more common for them to just be one layer of the pain. And here's another thing about trigger points: just about every symptom of pelvic pain can be caused by them! Vulvar burning, penile pain, vestibule burning, urethral burning, anal pain: trigger points in the pelvic floor and girdle muscles can be at the heart of each of these symptoms.

Whether too-tight muscles or trigger points or both are at play, when it's primarily caused by tightness, muscle pain is typically achy in nature; however, it *can* also be burny, especially when trigger points irritate nearby nerves. In addition, it tends to get worse as the day goes on. Commonly, pelvic MRIs or CT scans are ordered for patients with pelvic pain; however, while these tests can identify more sinister issues,

Table 3.1.   Myofascial Trigger Point Referral Patterns

Muscle	Referral Pattern
Rectus abdominis	Mid and low back and viscerosomatic symptoms
Iliopsoas	Paravertebral and anterior thigh
Quadratus lumborum	Iliac crest, outer thigh, buttock
Gluteus maximus	Sacrum, coccyx, buttock
Gluteus medius	Low back, sacrum, buttock, lateral hip/thigh
Adductors	Groin and inner thigh
Hamstrings	Gluteal fold, posterior thigh, popliteal fossa
Piriformis	Low back, buttock, posterior thigh
Obturator internus	Coccyx and posterior thigh, fullness in rectum or vaginal pain
Coccygeus	Coccyx, sacrum, rectum
Pubococcygeus	Coccyx, sacrum, rectum
Iliococcygeus	Coccyx, sacrum, rectum
Ischiocavernosus	Perineal aching
Bulbospongiosus	Dyspareunia/impotence, perineal pain with sitting
Transverse perineum	Dyspareunia
External anal sphincter	Diffuse ache, pain with bowel movements, constipation
Urinary sphincter	Urinary retention, perineal urge, frequency

Source: Pelvic Health and Rehabilitation Center

like tumors, they will not diagnose tight muscles or the existence of trigger points. The best way to identify either is through an intravaginal or intrarectal exam, which a pelvic floor PT will do.

CONNECTIVE TISSUE RESTRICTION

Restricted connective tissue is another common impairment involved in pelvic pain. Most people aren't aware of the role connective tissue can play in pain. Not many people who are in pain will say, "My connective tissue hurts!" The job of connective tissue is to support, connect, or separate different types of tissue and organs. Ligaments, tendons, and cartilage are all considered connective tissue. However, the type of connective tissue that we're interested in when it comes to pelvic pain is known as "loose connective tissue." Loose connective tissue is aptly named, because its fibers are randomly arranged, and there's lots of space between the cells, which makes it the ideal tissue for cushioning and protecting. (For the sake of brevity, even though we're referring specifically to "loose connective tissue," going forward we'll be using the term "connective tissue.") Besides surrounding blood vessels and nerves, one of the biggest jobs of connective tissue in the body is to attach the skin to the muscles.

Connective tissue can become restricted as a result of dysfunction in underlying muscle, nerves, joints, and organs. When we talk about connective tissue as it relates to pelvic pain, we're talking about tissue in areas from the navel to the knees, back and front, and in certain cases also above and below these areas. The connective tissue that plays the largest role in pelvic pain includes the tissue of the abdomen, the inner and outer thighs, the hips, the buttocks, the tissue over the pubic bone and sit bones, and the tissue around the anus. When the connective tissue that attaches the skin to the muscle becomes restricted (think thickened or dense), it can and does cause pain. The main reason is that it causes decreased blood flow to the area. On top of all that, it's hypothesized that restricted connective tissue can cause referred pain—pain to organs (think bladder in the case of pelvic pain). Local symptoms of connective tissue restriction when it comes to pelvic pain include hypersensitivity (intolerance to clothing), itching (anal or vulvar itching in the absence of infection), visual changes (redness and/or darkened tissue), and/or impaired integrity (splitting of tissue). The severity of connective tissue restriction ranges. For example, a patient may have moderate connective tissue restriction, so when he is standing, it doesn't bother him. But when he sits, he compresses the too-tight tissue, further restricting blood flow and causing pain. Without treatment his symptoms may progress from provoked pain when sitting to unprovoked standing pain. Also, often women with vulvar pain and pain with sex have restricted vulvar connective tissue. Indeed, when this tissue is manipulated in PT, they often report that it reproduces their pain with intercourse. (Being able to reproduce symptoms in this way is always a good sign. As a general rule of thumb, when we can reproduce symptoms, we can often get rid of them.) In addition, restricted connective tissue in the vulva can cause itching or burning and restricted connective tissue in the abdomen can contribute to abdominal pain.

Peripheral nerves are the nerves outside the brain and spinal cord. When people think of peripheral nerves in relation to pelvic pain, they typically think of the pudendal nerve, but quite a few peripheral nerves can contribute to symptoms of pelvic pain. See table 3.2 for the names of these nerves as well as information on the areas they innervate.

Peripheral nerves can be injured or irritated for a number of different reasons. For one thing, they can become compressed. Nerves can become compressed by organs, scar tissue, behaviors/postures (sitting), activity (riding a bike or a horse), or placement of a foreign object (mesh). A particular kind of compression occurs when a nerve becomes "entrapped." For its part, entrapment occurs when a nerve's mobility is severely limited because it's stuck in tissue or some sort of anatomical tunnel, causing it to be severely compressed. Nerves can become entrapped by scar tissue, a foreign object (mesh), or an anatomic anomaly (someone could be born with a nerve that's entangled in a ligament, for instance). In the case of the pudendal nerve, for example, the two ligaments that surround the nerve can create a space that is too tight for the nerve, causing problems. In addition, nerves can get injured by stretch mechanisms such as a vaginal delivery, constipation, or deep and heavy squats. Lastly, infection can cause a nerve to become irritated. It's important to understand that an irritated nerve can cause dysfunction to whatever tissue it supplies. Muscles, organs, and skin can all be affected. *So how can a peripheral nerve issue translate into the symptoms of pelvic pain?* One example involves hernia surgery. During the

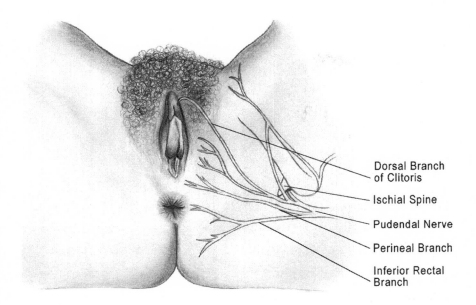

Dorsal Branch of Clitoris

Ischial Spine

Pudendal Nerve

Perineal Branch

Inferior Rectal Branch

Figure 3.2. Pudendal nerve and its branches. *Source: Pelvic Health and Rehabilitation Center*

surgery, the ilioinguinal nerve, which is located in the abdominal wall, can be affected and create penile and scrotal pain. Another involves impairment of the pudendal nerve, which can create burning vaginal or clitoral pain in women or penile, scrotal, or perineum pain in men. Lastly, the posterior femoral cutaneous nerve, which is located in the thigh, can cause pain with sitting and/or perineum pain. In addition to the major nerves of the pelvic floor, loads of tiny, superficial nerve branches can play a role in pelvic pain, in areas such as the vulva/vestibule, for instance. Indeed, vulvar/vestibule pain can be caused by an increase in nerve fiber density in the area. Nerve pain in the pelvis is typically sharp, shooting, stabbing, knife-like, burning, or itching anywhere in the distribution of the impacted nerves. Impaired nerves can also cause numbness.

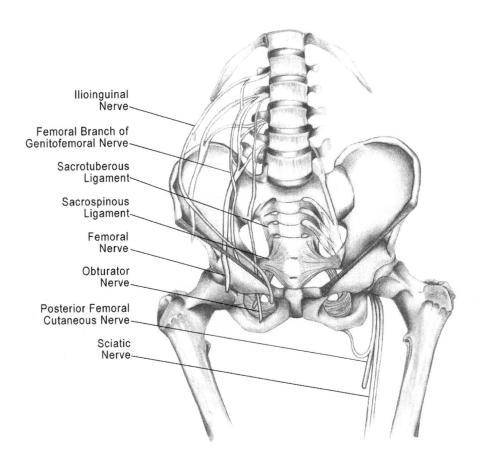

Ilioinguinal Nerve

Femoral Branch of Genitofemoral Nerve

Sacrotuberous Ligament

Sacrospinous Ligament

Femoral Nerve

Obturator Nerve

Posterior Femoral Cutaneous Nerve

Sciatic Nerve

Figure 3.3.   Peripheral nerves of the pelvis. *Source: Pelvic Health and Rehabilitation Center*

HOW THE CENTRAL NERVOUS SYSTEM FITS IN

With persistent pain, whether it's pelvic pain, knee pain, or back pain, we cannot ignore the role of the central nervous system (the brain and the spinal cord), because it's always involved. *What is that role?* Being in pain, including pelvic pain, can actually change how the brain and spinal cord receive input and produce symptoms. After tissues have healed from an injury, which is typically around 12 weeks, the brain can still create the *pain symptoms* of the initial injury, even though there is no longer a problem with the tissue. *So why bring this up now?* All the

Table 3.2.   Pelvic Nerves and the Structures They Supply

Nerve	Innervation
Pudendal	External genitalia, skin of the perineum and around the anus
Ilioinguinal	In men: skin over the root of the penis and upper part of the scrotum; in women: skin over the mons pubis and labia majora
Genitofemoral	Upper anterior thigh, skin of anterior scrotum in men, and mons pubis in women
Iliohypogastric	Skin over the lateral buttocks and above the pubis
Posterior femoral cutaneous	Posterior surface of thigh and leg and skin of perineum
Sciatic	Posterior portion of the thigh
Cluneal	Skin of the buttocks

Source: Pelvic Health and Rehabilitation Center

neuromuscular impairments we discussed above actually have the potential to modify the way our brain and spinal cord work, thereby, and unknown to the person dealing with the symptom-causing impairments, creating a perception of pain that's out of sync with the impairment or that hangs around once the impairment is cleared up. Specifically, someone with persistent pain can get to a place where they're actually having more pain with less or even no provocation. This phenomenon is called "central sensitization." Before we go into any more detail about how the nervous system can become sensitized in this way, we first want to talk a little about how pain works, including what it means to have "persistent pain" versus its counterpart, "acute pain."

Pain is a protective mechanism generated by the brain in response to a perceived threat, like burning your hand on the stove, which creates pain from the burned tissue. Oftentimes the degree of pain experienced is actually not directly in proportion to tissue damage. Consider this: a paper cut produces very little tissue damage yet can cause a lot of pain. Conversely, a soldier can get shot in battle yet not realize he's injured until he's off the battlefield. In some cases, pain may not be associated with tissue damage at all. For example, amputees may experience phantom limb pain in tissue that no longer exists, because the part of the brain that corresponded to the amputated limb can still generate the sensation of pain, even after the limb is gone. Plus, pain relies on context. For instance, athletes involved in vigorous sports ignore impacts that would send most of us screaming because it's all part of the game, and in that context the pain is expected and not threatening. "Catastrophic thinking," which is basically when a person ruminates about worst-case outcomes, can actually make pain worse. However, knowing pain is generated by the brain rather than by damaged tissues does not mean that pain is "all in your head" and should be ignored or dismissed. In fact, knowing that pain is the body's alarm system actually highlights the importance of treating it before the alarm system becomes wonky, overreacting to every perceived threat. So "acute pain" actually helps you avoid danger or more tissue damage. Persistent pain happens when pain occurs either in the complete absence of tissue damage or after the tissue damage has healed. (Persistent pain is typically considered pain lasting six months or more.) Central sensitization is the term used to describe that wonky pain loop. A sensitized nervous system is responsible for persistent pain. And what's happening is either the pain itself or other factors have modified the way the central nervous system works, so that a person actually becomes more sensitive and gets *more pain* with *less provocation or even no provocation*. This phenomenon involves changes to the central nervous system, in particular the brain and the spinal cord. So a sensitized nervous system not only makes people more sensitive to things that *should* hurt, but also to things that should not, like ordinary touch and pressure, for example. Patients tell us things like "my husband lightly touched my stomach and I jumped five feet" or "touching a cold floor with bare feet actually hurts." Other common examples of a sensitized nervous system that we see with our patients are intolerance to tight jeans and/or underwear and pain with sitting. In addition, when a sensitized nervous system is at play, any pain the person experiences might fade more slowly than it would in someone who doesn't have a sensitized nervous system. For example, a woman, let's call her Cynthia, who has had anal pain for a few years, and who has a sensitized nervous system as one element of her pain, gets a fairly normal vaginal yeast infection. In most cases, this kind of infection is treated with medication, clears up, and the pain stops. Life goes on. But in Cynthia's case, this little infection jacks up her anal pain (even though the infection has nothing to do with her anus), and the vaginal pain that is a symptom of the infection, instead of clearing up as soon as the infection does, lasts for weeks afterward. So in essence, a sensitized nervous system can cause a person to have more pain and for longer from something fairly benign versus someone whose nervous system is not sensitized. As providers who treat a persistent pain syndrome, we have to consider with each patient the role the central nervous system plays in their pain. Plus, as we've already mentioned, patients with pelvic pain are often initially misdiagnosed and don't get on the path to appropriate treatment right away. Oftentimes it can take six months to a year for them to get on that road, setting them up to develop a sensitized nervous system as one layer of their pain. We want to make it clear that we're not saying every person who has had pelvic pain for six months or more will develop a sensitized nervous system as a pain driver. That is simply not what we've seen in our years of treating pelvic pain. Time and again we have treated patients who have had symptoms for six months to a year and beyond, and after their tissue impairments are adequately treated, their pain has gone away. What we *are* saying is that with pelvic pain, providers must consider whether a patient's central nervous system is playing a role, and to what extent. And if they do believe the patient's pain has a strong central nervous system component, take steps to ensure that this layer of pain is dealt with, because doing so is every bit as important as working out a trigger point or loosening restricted connective tissue when it comes to a patient's recovery. That's why in chapter 5, we discuss how the central nervous system fits into our treatment approach and in chapter 6 we discuss other options for treating it.

In this chapter, we've taken a close look at exactly how neuromuscular impairments of the pelvic floor actually translate into the variety of symptoms associated with pelvic pain. A major takeaway is that these impairments can kick off a vicious cycle. A tight muscle causes a trigger point to form. A trigger point causes a nearby nerve to become irritated. An irritated nerve causes surrounding muscle to tighten, causing connective tissue restriction. These impairments cause pain, alerting the brain that something is wrong and ultimately changing the way the brain processes pain. A person becomes anxious, further increasing their pain. A vicious cycle has been set in motion. That's why in the next section of the book we will explore exactly how to go about breaking that cycle, beginning with a basic question: I have pelvic pain; now what do I do?

II

Getting on the Road to Healing

4

I HAVE PELVIC PAIN. WHAT DO I DO NOW?

Beth, a 31-year-old woman, woke up one morning with vulvar and vaginal burning. Assuming she had a yeast infection, a regular affliction for her, she self-treated with the usual over-the-counter medication. Three boxes of OTC medication later, she was still in pain. It was time to see a doctor. She made an appointment with her gynecologist. A barrage of tests came back negative. Fear set in. Seemingly overnight, things she had taken for granted like sitting, driving, and even wearing underwear and jeans became difficult because they exacerbated her pain. Sex was out of the question. So Beth did what millions of people with a health problem do: she logged on to the Internet. Googling "vaginal burning" and "vulvar burning" landed her in an online chat room for women diagnosed with "pudendal neuralgia." After reading horror story after horror story, her fear turned to terror and she was left wondering: *"Now what do I do?"*

Beth is one of many men and women with pelvic pain in the United States (and abroad) asking that question. We know this for a fact, because each day at our clinics, we get dozens of calls and e-mails, all different versions of the same question. As we've discussed in previous chapters, it's only in recent years that meaningful strides have been made in the understanding of chronic pain in general. And although there has been a momentum in research to study chronic pain, and pelvic pain specifically, it's still early days on both fronts. Therefore, when diagnosing and treating pelvic pain, there simply isn't a large body of time- *and* research-tested treatment options available for providers to draw from. As a result, it can still be difficult for pelvic pain sufferers to get an appropriate diagnosis and treatment. That's why we're devoting an entire chapter to providing a road map for patients to get on the right treatment path. Specifically, this chapter details three steps for patients to get on that path. They are:

1. Getting educated about pelvic pain.
2. Finding the right doctor.
3. Finding the right physical therapist (PT).

GETTING EDUCATED

Even though it can be a slippery slope, the Internet is a good place for those with pelvic pain to begin their education about the condition. Thankfully, today there are some fantastic pelvic pain–related blogs and online support groups. (See appendix A for a complete list of online resources that we have vetted and highly recommend.) Our advice to go online for information comes with a caveat, however. The Internet can be a terrifying place for a person in pain. Horror stories abound. So it's important to keep in mind that the majority of folks on the Internet are the ones struggling to get better; therefore, a disproportionate number of people online are not getting better versus those who are. Also, it's important for those who turn to the Internet for information to remember to *not* believe everything they read and to always consider the source. And even though their symptoms might seem exactly like someone else's that they read about, the underlying causes and circumstances are almost always going to be different, so what worked for one may or may not work for another. Bottom line: turn to the Internet to become an informed patient who can advocate for yourself, but always pay attention to the source of the information. Take what you need and leave the rest. And DO NOT linger in chat rooms filled with hard luck stories. Research shows that fear and anxiety absolutely, positively exacerbate pain. Lastly, do not use the Internet to glom on to a diagnosis. For instance, we regularly have people call, write in, and come to our clinics convinced that they have pudendal neuralgia or pudendal nerve entrapment because they've read about these particular diagnoses on-line.

FINDING A DOCTOR

When it comes to pelvic pain treatment, it's important to see a doctor to rule out infection or any other more serious pathology. But besides being able to rule out a serious pathology, a physician plays an important role in an interdisciplinary treatment approach to pelvic pain, namely, to manage any necessary medications and/or treat contributing factors, such as endometriosis, a Bartholin's abscess, dermatological issues, or hormone imbalances, just to name a few. Only a handful of physicians specialize in pelvic pain in the United States. Many people don't have the resources to travel to see one of these specialists, and as we'll explain, unless one of the few pelvic pain specialists is local to you, it's ultimately not necessary for your physician to be a specialist. Plus, it's important to remember that treating pelvic pain, more often than not, is going to be a longer-term process that involves PT. So at the end of the day, it makes sense to find a local physician to join your treatment team. The good news is, contrary to what most patients believe, a local physician, whether a gynecologist, urologist, or primary care physician, will more often than not be able to offer therapeutic options *even if they are not a pelvic pain specialist*. However, because many patients don't understand this treatment model from the outset, they're disappointed after they see a doctor because they expected to leave the appointment with a definitive diagnosis, treatment, and cure. We're hoping that the information provided in this chapter will spare patients that disappointment by explaining the role a local physician typically plays in an inter-disciplinary treatment plan.

Typically the physician a female patient will visit is a gynecologist, unless her symptoms are mainly urological, in which case she'll see a urologist. Male patients usually start out going to a primary care physician, who may then refer them to a urologist. For the most part, treatment options these physicians can offer include medication to manage pain/other symptoms, topical creams, and/or possibly some sort of injection. (We will be going into much greater detail about these and other treatment options in chapter 8.) In addition, the physician can offer a referral to a pelvic floor PT as well as a pain management doctor.

So how do you know if a physician is a good fit to join your treatment team? Our advice is to explain your symptoms to the doctor, and if he/she looks perplexed or suggests a treatment that you've already tried, but that didn't work in the past, it's fair to ask the doctor if he/she feels comfortable treating your symptoms or if he/she has had experience with similar patients in the past. If the doctor says no or you are uncomfortable, then we recommend that you move on to the next doctor. Basically, you want a doctor who has an interest in learning about pelvic pain and with whom you can communicate comfortably. Another piece of advice is for you to share articles with the doctor that you believe pertain to your symptoms. (See appendix A for a list of blog posts from our blog and/or articles that may be appropriate to take to your doctor.)

When should you visit one of the few pelvic pain specialists practicing today? If you believe you have reached a plateau with your treatment plan, it might be worth seeing a pelvic pain specialist for a consultation to help modify, improve, or redirect your treatment in consultation with your local providers. But you always want to exhaust your local resources before traveling to a specialist and keep your local provider in the loop if you do. An exception to this rule is the few cases where a specialist is truly needed because of their expertise in a particular area, such as actual pudendal nerve entrapment, Tarlov cysts, or mesh removal.

At what point is it advisable to add a pain management doctor to your treatment team? Our thinking is that anytime a patient is going to take medication as part of his/her treatment plan, it's best for a pain management doctor to act as the prescribing physician, as medication management for persistent pain is their area of expertise. And bear in mind that a pain management doctor does not need to have expertise treating pelvic pain to be a valuable member of a treatment team. These physicians have experience treating all types of pain. We'd like to include the same caveat for visiting a pain management doctor that we brought up for a visit to a local physician. The pain management doctor's role in treatment is to help patients manage their symptoms, not to eradicate the problem. Besides asking your local physician if he/she has a trusted referral, a good resource for finding a pain management doctor is the International Association for the Study of Pain, a medical organization devoted to pain.

FINDING A PT

As already discussed in previous chapters, almost all pelvic pain syndromes involve some kind of neuromuscular issue, that is, a problem with the muscles, nerves, and connective tissue of the pelvic floor and adjacent areas. A PT is the medical provider who has the best understanding of the neuromuscular system and is therefore best equipped to treat it. It's important to see a PT who specializes in treating the pelvic floor. A decade ago qualified pelvic floor PTs were few and far between. Fast-forward to today. Marked progress has been made in pelvic pain PT education with more and more educational opportunities available to PTs. For example, when we graduated from PT school more than 15 years ago, we were not aware that pelvic floor rehabilitation was an available career path. Today PTs are graduating with an awareness that this specialty exists. Furthermore, today many postgraduate classes on pelvic pain treatment are available to PTs. In addition, medical institutions around the country have caught on to the demand for pelvic pain rehabilitation and have opened interdisciplinary pelvic pain clinics, many of which include on-staff pelvic floor PTs.

So how do you go about finding a knowledgeable and qualified pelvic floor PT? Fortunately, they are out there, and below is a list of resources for connecting with them:

American Physical Therapy Association

The APTA is a professional association for PTs in the United States. On its website, the organization offers a searchable database of "women's health" PTs. While pelvic pain does not discriminate between the sexes, the APTA is still working to iron out this discrepancy. In the meantime, many of the PTs listed in the APTA's "women's health" locator treat both men and women. You can find the APTA's women's health locator at www.womenshealthapta.org/find-a-physical-therapist/index.cfm.

Pelvic Floor Physical Therapy Classes

One great way to find a pelvic floor PT is to get in touch with the organizations that are teaching postgraduate courses in pelvic floor PT in cities around the United States. We teach such a class, so feel free to contact us, and if we know of a PT in your area that we are comfortable recommending, we will be more than happy to do so. Check out our website at www.pelvicpainrehab.com for our contact information. The Herman & Wallace Pelvic Rehabilitation Institute also teaches a variety of postgraduate pelvic floor PT courses. So a patient could contact the faculty members of Herman & Wallace and ask for a PT recommendation as well. You can find the Herman & Wallace website at http://hermanwallace.com.

The International Pelvic Pain Society

The IPPS has a "find a provider" option on its website at www.pelvicpain.org that includes a search for PTs.

Happy Pelvis

Happy Pelvis, a Yahoo support group, is a good resource for PT recommendations. The group was started specifically to support pelvic pain patients through the physical therapy process. Today Happy Pelvis has hundreds of active members who are always willing to recommend PTs. In addition, there is a searchable list of pelvic pain PTs in the group's archives. You can find Happy Pelvis at http://groups.yahoo.com/neo/groups/happypelvis/info.

Pelvic Pain Bloggers

The bloggers we include in our list of blogs in appendix A may be able to recommend a qualified PT. In fact, many of the bloggers are PTs themselves.

#pelvicmafia

The PTs in this Twitter group are always happy to recommend a PT if they can.

Above are all great resources to help you find a pelvic floor PT in your area. However, unfortunately, a few regions of the country have no qualified pelvic floor PTs . . . yet. *What do you do if you live in one of these areas?* Though it's not an ideal situation, patients will travel to see a qualified pelvic floor PT for a period of intensive treatment. *What do you do if you have to travel out of town for treatment but need it on a long-term basis, as so many pelvic pain patients ultimately do?* Some of our out-of-town patients arrange for a local PT who is not yet qualified to treat pelvic pain, but is willing to learn, to travel with them so we can show him/her how to best treat them, or they bring along their significant other to learn how to administer certain treatment techniques. The good news is that compared to even five years ago, the number of PTs treating pelvic pain has significantly increased and continues to do so thanks to new educational opportunities for PTs interested in pursuing this specialty. Plus, it's important to bear in mind that while treatment with a qualified pelvic floor PT is often an important component of an interdisciplinary treatment plan, there are several other avenues, as we will cover in great detail in upcoming chapters, which, when combined, can lead to recovery.

QUESTIONS TO ASK A POTENTIAL PT

Once you zero in on a PT, you can ask him or her a handful of questions to make sure he or she is a good fit. We've included that list of questions below.

1. *What is your approach to treating pelvic pain?* What you're looking for here is an approach that includes manual therapy techniques (connective tissue manipulation, trigger point therapies, joint mobilization, and nerve glides), delivered internally through the vagina or anus and externally to the pelvic floor and adjacent areas, such as the abdomen, hips, and inner/outer thighs. Other techniques used to treat pelvic pain include home exercises, neuromuscular reeducation, and central nervous system strate-

gies for decreasing pain. (The next chapter is a complete over-view of pelvic pain PT and will give you a much clearer under-standing of physical therapy techniques used to treat pelvic pain.)

2. *How long are your treatment sessions?* Treating pelvic pain can be time consuming because of the number of structures that are often involved in a pelvic pain syndrome. In an ideal setting, a treatment session should be an hour-long, one-on-one treatment session with the PT. Due to current health care constraints, how-ever, this may not be possible, and the treatment times may be shorter.

3. *What percentage of your patients have pelvic pain?* In addition to pelvic pain, pelvic floor PTs are also trained to treat urinary and fecal incontinence, prepartum and postpartum dysfunction, and pelvic organ prolapse. While all these issues involve the pelvic floor, treatment for them is very different than treatment for pelvic pain. Therefore, it's important to find a PT with a specific interest in pelvic pain under the umbrella of pelvic floor disor-ders.

MOLLY'S STORY

One month after my thirty-second birthday, I woke up in excruciating pain—it was as if someone had set me on fire while I slept—the focal point of my pain was the left side of my vulva, but I also had extreme vaginal and urethral burning. My first thought was that I had either a yeast or bladder infection. I had just moved to California three weeks before, so I had to find a doctor on the fly and hope for the best. Dr. Number One took several tests and sent me home with a goody bag full of creams, suppositories, and other meds. None of the remedies worked, and all the tests came back negative. From there I began to see the doctor regularly in an effort to get to the bottom of my pain. After about the third visit, he told me he didn't know what was causing my pain, but that my pelvic floor muscles were tight. He diagnosed me with vulvodynia and recommended that I see a "vulvodynia specialist" as well as a PT. At this point I was in a full-on state of panic—it felt like I had a pile of burning coals inside me—it hurt to sit, it hurt to stand, it hurt to urinate, sex was out of the question, I wasn't sleeping or eating—I was truly in agony. In my state of anxiety I couldn't figure out how on earth a PT would be able to help me—wasn't a PT for a person who had broken his leg or been in a car accident? I honestly didn't understand how a PT could heal the kind of pain I was in. So I put the info away and concentrated on getting an appointment with Dr. Vulvodynia Specialist. To my utter dismay, his solution was to give me Capsaicin treatments, which consisted of me applying cream made from the hottest, reddest peppers on the planet to my already-on-fire vulva daily. Ugh, no. Check, please! After this incident I sought out two more opinions—one doctor, we'll call him Dr. Google, actually googled "vulvodynia" right in front of me. After scanning the info he came up with, he said, "Yep, you have vulvodynia." He also added that there was no way my pelvic floor muscles were too tight, and that getting PT for relief would be a waste of time. The next doctor told me that nothing whatsoever was wrong with me—great news, except for the part where I remained in terrible pain. Not long after, there came a day when I decided if I had to live life in such horrible pain, I'd rather not (just a little aside here—no one is more against death than me, so for me to even be thinking this way was incredible). That day I did what you do when you don't know what to do; I called my mom, and she told me to go straight to the hospital. At the time, a trip to the emergency room sounded like a wonderful idea to me. Truth be told, I had been harboring this fantasy of lying in a hospital bed surrounded by a team of doctors whose mission it was to figure out exactly what was wrong with me, and then cure me. But once again my hopes for getting to the bottom of my pain were dashed. It took a couple of doctors and an intern or two to tell me nothing showed up on any of the tests they ran on me, and they simply didn't know what was causing my pain. The day after the emergency room fiasco, I decided to call the PT that Dr. Number One had told me about and make an appointment. I was burned out on doctors, but I didn't want to give up. At least seeing a PT would keep me in the game. And that's when things began to turn around for me. The PT I saw was Stephanie. After working on the external connective tissue restrictions I had, Stephanie began to work on me internally. About five minutes into the session she found what she described as a "pea-size lump" on the left side of my vaginal wall. She referred me to a pelvic surgeon, who diagnosed me with a Bartholin's abscess. I was overjoyed that someone had finally found "the reason" for my pain. However, my happiness was short-lived, as two months after the surgery to remove the cyst, I was still in pain. Back to PT I went. What Stephanie found was that many of my pelvic floor muscles were tight, including the muscles surrounding my urethra, and that the muscle adjacent to where the cyst had been was riddled with trigger points. Apparently the muscle guarding I had done for the past year to "protect" my painful tissue had resulted in muscle tightening and trigger points. In addition to that, I had a great deal of connective tissue restriction on my inner thighs, sit bone area, abdomen, and bony pelvis. There was a lot of work to do. After six months of regular PT with Stephanie, I reached a place where I was about 90% pain-free. I do have urethral symptoms that fluctuate depending on how active I am, and the occasional bout of pain with sitting. But I manage both symptoms, and neither interferes with my ability to live my life to the fullest. I have pain-free sex, wear jeans, do yoga, and exercise. Recovery was a hard road, but once I got on the right path, with lots of patience and persistence I did get better, and if you're a patient reading this, you will too.

DIRECT ACCESS TO PHYSICAL THERAPY

While we recommend that patients see a physician prior to starting PT for all the above-mentioned reasons, there are situations where going straight to a pelvic floor PT without seeing a doctor first is an option. Indeed, at the time of this book's writing, all 50 states, including the District of Columbia, have some form of "direct access" law in place. Direct access is just what it sounds like. It allows patients to have direct access to PTs without a physician referral or prescription. However, some states have provisions tied to treatment without a physician referral, such as a time or visit limit. For example, in California, one of the states where we practice, after either 12 visits or 45 days, whichever comes first, patients must visit their doctor to have him/her sign off on the PT's plan of care, among other provisions. The direct access laws are often in flux, so if you have any questions about how the law applies in your specific state, we recommend that you contact the American Physical Therapy Association, the national professional organization for physical therapy. The organization publishes updated news on the direct access laws on its site at www.apta.org/directaccess, and you can contact the APTA directly as a consumer with questions at consu-mer@apta.org.

We believe patients can benefit from the direct access laws in a few specific situations. For example, it's not uncommon for patients to have long wait times before getting in to see their doctors. In this situation, it makes sense to start PT while they are waiting for the appointment, because then treatment can begin as soon as possible and the PT can communicate his/her findings to the physician. In addition, the PT can help the patient organize the information he/she will communicate to the doctor and help him/her formulate questions to ask during the appointment. Another example of the benefits of direct access is when a patient has seen a PT in the past and is just going in for a "tune-up" or because of symptom recurrence. A final example is when a patient has been to a physician/physicians who have ruled out other pathologies but did not know to refer the patient to PT. Patients can share their re-search regarding pelvic floor PT with their doctor and discuss their progress with him or her along the way. In these situations, physicians are often relieved that the patient has a solution when he or she may be at a loss. We have treated many patients in the past who found us without a physician referral. Typically we advise these patients to in-clude at least one doctor in their treatment plan, and we help coordi-nate communication with this provider. This is actually how Beth, whose story kicked off the chapter, got to our office. After not getting answers from the doctors she saw, and encouraged by the members of the Happy Pelvis online group mentioned above, she made an appoint-ment to see Liz. Fortunately Beth's impairments were pretty straight-forward. She had severe tightness and trigger points in her pelvic floor as well as inner thigh connective tissue restrictions. After about five months of weekly manual internal and external PT, Beth was nearly pain-free.

It is our hope that this chapter has clearly explained the important first steps people dealing with pelvic pain must take to begin down the path toward healing. Armed from the outset with the knowledge that the path to recovery will be different from what they've experienced when seeking treatment for other conditions can remove much of the anxiety and frustration from the endeavor, leaving them to focus on what's important: getting better. Coming up in chapter 5, we're going to talk about a major component in the path toward recovery: pelvic floor physical therapy.

5

PELVIC PAIN PT: IN THE TREATMENT ROOM

HOW EXACTLY DOES A PHYSICAL THERAPIST TREAT PELVIC PAIN?

This is probably the most frequently asked question we get from patients and providers. It's understandable, as most people's experience with PT involves orthopedic PT following a surgery or injury, so it's hard for them to imagine how the physical therapy they're familiar with translates to treatment for pelvic pain. That's why in this chapter we're going to take you into the treatment room and show you exactly how we as pelvic floor PTs evaluate a patient and assess what is behind his/her symptoms. In addition, we take you through two important steps we take as we develop a treatment plan for patients—setting goals for treatment and coordinating with a patient's interdisciplinary treatment team. Lastly, we'll end the chapter with an explanation of where a sensitized nervous system fits into our treatment approach as well as a discussion of some specific issues that men with pelvic pain face as they navigate treatment.

EVALUATION: GETTING A HISTORY

At our clinic, treatment for pelvic pain begins with an evaluation. When we evaluate patients, our goal is to identify the contributing factors and impairments behind their pain. The bulk of the evaluation takes place at the first appointment, but it's not uncommon for it to take two to three appointments for us to get a complete picture of what's behind a patient's symptoms. Because no two cases of pelvic pain are the same, each patient evaluation is going to be different, but there are enough common notes that we can give you a general overview of how we evaluate a patient beginning with the first appointment. During the first appointment, the process of putting together the pieces of the puzzle of a patient's pain begins with a discussion of his/her history. Here we put our detective hats on and ask a series of questions about the history and onset of the patient's pain. Among the questions we ask are *What do you think caused your pain? Describe your symptoms? How long have you had symptoms? What exacerbates and alleviates your symptoms? What activities do your symptoms limit? What providers have you seen? What past treatments have you had, what has helped, and what has not? Describe the severity of your symptoms?* (For a complete list of the questions we ask our patients during their first appointment, see appendix B.) In addition to questions about the pain, we ask specific questions about urinary, bowel, and sexual function. For example, we ask patients if they experience urinary urgency, constipation, or pain with penetration or after ejaculation. Commonly the PT evaluation is the first time a patient has been asked these questions. And while some are surprised that we're asking them questions of such a personal nature, more often than not, they're relieved to finally be telling a medical provider things like how much sex hurts, that they're having trouble reaching orgasm, that they have to use their finger to assist in a bowel movement, or that they notice their urine stream doesn't sound as forceful as their counterpart's in a public restroom. This Q&A portion of the first appointment begins the process of gathering clues that we'll use to figure out why a patient is having pain and what needs to be done to address it. It also gives us the road map we use for the next part of the appointment—the hands-on examination. A patient's list of symptoms can be quite long, so during the interview, we work to suss out the symptoms that are the most bothersome for them. Because time is limited, we'll attack these symptoms first during the hands-on exam. What's more, information we get from patients at this point will guide us in approaching that exam. For example, as discussed in chapter 3, people suffering from persistent pain often develop a sensitized nervous system. This has to be considered before the examination, because it actually dictates our approach. For instance, we'll move more slowly through the exam, or we may not use certain evaluation techniques that have the potential to aggravate a sensitized nervous system. (We'll discuss more on how the central nervous system fits into our treatment approach below.) By the time the interview has come to a close, we've formulated a plan for the upcoming exam. After discussing it with the patient and asking if he/she has any questions, we leave the room to allow the patient to disrobe from the waist down, drape themselves, and get comfortable on the treatment table. From there the exam begins.

EVALUATION: HANDS-ON EXAMINATION

The goal of the evaluation exam is to begin uncovering a patient's symptom-causing impairments. In addition, we continue our search for all the factors contributing to a patient's pain. As already mentioned, during the exam we focus first on the areas we believe are causing the patient's most painful symptoms. But in general, during this hands-on portion of the exam, we're looking for the three common neuromuscular impairments we discussed in chapter 3: connective tissue restrictions, internal and external muscle impairments (too-tight muscles and/or trigger points), and peripheral nerve dysfunction. In addition, we're also going to check for any anatomical/biomechanical abnormalities (as discussed in chapter 2) by observing a combination of things, like posture and how the patient walks.

External Exam

We begin the exam externally. External structures we examine for possible impairments include the abdomen, hip muscles, inner/outer thighs, low back, and the sacroiliac and hip joints. When beginning the external exam, we'll always focus first on the structures we believe are the most relevant to the patient's symptoms. For example, if a patient complains of tailbone pain, we'll first examine his sacroiliac joint and the soft tissue around his tailbone, followed by a rectal examination. That's because impairments in these areas are commonly behind tailbone pain. Less important to this particular patient would be an evaluation of the abdominal wall, as it's typically not a generator of tailbone pain. In general, among other things, we're on the hunt for connective tissue restrictions, trigger points, or nerve dysfunction.

A major component of the external exam is our search for any possible connective tissue restrictions. Restricted connective tissue can cause symptoms such as pain with sitting or vulvar burning. As you'll recall from previous chapters, when we talk about connective tissue as it relates to pelvic pain, we're talking about tissue in the areas from the navel to the knees, back and front, and in certain cases, above and below these areas. Happy connective tissue is mobile, uniform in its density, and does not produce pain when touched. Restricted connective tissue is thick or "gummed up" and lacks mobility or is "sticky," and when examined, the patient will typically feel discomfort. Because of the referred pain patterns that can occur with connective tissue restriction, however, this discomfort may actually be felt elsewhere. Indeed, patients are often surprised when an area of connective tissue triggers their symptoms in another area. For instance, a female patient whose main complaint is pain with intercourse may have connective tissue restrictions in her abdomen around her belly button. While we're examining this area, it may cause vulvar discomfort or reproduce the vulvar pain she feels with intercourse. If we find that a patient's connective tissue is restricted in any of the areas we examine, we basically "pinch roll" the affected tissue below the skin and above the muscle between the thumb and four other fingers, with both hands. This is commonly referred to as "skin rolling." This technique is used to both evaluate and treat the tissue. What we're checking for when we evaluate connective tissue is how well it moves, its density, and its sensitivity. Treatment is aimed at loosening the tissue to improve blood flow, decrease thickness, and restore mobility. When tissue is restricted, manipulating it typically causes a sharp sensation and may even cause soreness or bruising in the days following treatment. As the patient's tissue normalizes over a series of appointments, however, the treatment becomes less painful.

Typically, after we examine a patient externally for connective tissue restrictions, we move on to areas that may harbor trigger points. External trigger points can be involved in a slew of different pelvic pain symptoms. For instance, if a patient has pain with sitting, we may find a trigger point in her obturator internus muscle, one of the pelvic girdle muscles that can be accessed externally. The majority of pelvic floor

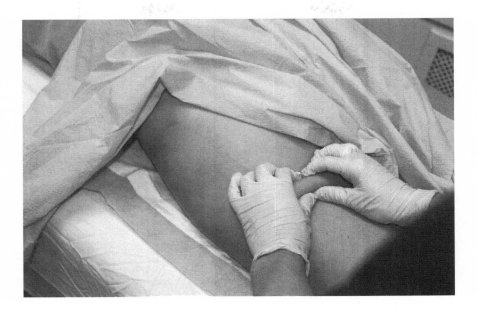

Figure 5.1.   Connective tissue manipulation of the back of the thigh. *Source: Pelvic Health and Rehabilitation Center*

muscles can not be accessed externally, so for the most part, when we're examining a patient for external trigger points, we're examining the muscles attached to the outside of the pelvis, such as all the gluteal muscles, the hamstrings, and the abdominal muscles. When we find a trigger point (whether externally or internally), the patient will typically feel a sharp, stabbing pain. Palpation of the trigger point may also cause referred pain or reproduce one of his symptoms. (It's always a good thing when we can reproduce a patient's symptoms. That's because typically, if we can reproduce it, we can treat it.) For example, when we palpate a trigger point in the perineum of a male patient, it may reproduce the "golf ball" sensation he feels in his perineum when he sits. To us, a trigger point feels like a lentil, small and hard to the touch. In addition, it may twitch when compressed, and it often feels hotter than the surrounding tissue. We as PTs can use a variety of manual techniques to "release" (get rid of) a trigger point. Sometimes a trigger point can be successfully released in one treatment session, but more often than not, it takes place over multiple PT appointments. Other times, before we can get a trigger point to disappear, we must also work with the patient to clear up any ongoing contributing factors that caused the trigger point to form in the first place, like postural issues, for example.

Our next course of action in the external exam is to check for any impaired nerve mobility and/or nerve sensitivity. We use a few different techniques to evaluate and treat peripheral nerves. For example, we palpate, or lightly touch, peripheral nerves to determine whether they are involved in a patient's symptoms. If a nerve is tender when palpated, that's a clue that it may be part of the problem. Also, when appropriate, we can test whether the nerve has healthy mobility by moving the patient's extremities. For example, we'll bring the patient's knee toward his/her chest while gauging the nerve's reaction. Another way to test the nerve's mobility is to manipulate the connective tissue or muscles surrounding it. If a nerve has normal mobility, neither of these tests should cause pain or discomfort. If there is pain or discomfort, this is another clue that the nerve is likely involved. If a nerve *is* found to have impaired mobility or sensitivity, we use a number of different treatment strategies to resolve the muscle, tissue, and joint impairments contributing to the dysfunction. These treatment techniques involve manual therapy, exercise, and joint mobilizations.

Anatomical/Biomechanical Abnormalities

As we discussed in detail in chapter 2, a number of structural/biomechanical issues can play a role in pelvic pain. To review, some of the main ones are hip labral tears, sacroiliac joint dysfunction, leg length discrepancy, spine dysfunction, motor coordination issues, and dysfunctional posture. In the first evaluation appointment, if appropriate, we will work to figure out if any structural/biomechanical issues are driving the patient's pain. However, when evaluating a patient for structural/biomechanical abnormalities, the line from impairment to symptom is not always as direct or obvious as with the other impairment groups, such as the defined pain patterns associated with trigger points. For example, say a patient has a symptom of pain in the tailbone and anus with sitting or transitioning from a standing to a sitting position. On the surface it would make sense to look for trigger points or connective tissue restrictions in the area as the culprits. But a structural/biomechanical abnormality could actually be at play, such as sacroiliac joint dysfunction (an SI joint that is "out of alignment") that is altering the mobility of certain branches of the pudendal nerve. Another challenge in connecting any structural/biomechanical abnormality to a patient's symptoms involves spine pathology. Spine pathology is often associated with weakness of the core and the small muscles of the back. If these muscles are weak, the muscles of the pelvic floor will have to overcompensate to provide stability, especially during complex movements, like playing sports or lifting. So say a patient has a disc herniation in his low back that causes him low back pain. If this patient continues to play sports, despite his back issues, some of his pelvic girdle muscles, such as his hip external rotators (obturator internus and piriformis), are going to overcompensate to give him stability during the activities. As a result, these muscles could become too tight or develop trigger points, causing the patient pelvic pain such as pain with sitting or tailbone pain. Assessing patients for any structural/biomechanical abnormalities is especially important if their history reveals things like he/she had a fall prior to the onset of pain or he/she has long-standing orthopedic issues. But it's less relevant for other patients, such as the patient who developed pelvic pain as a result of numerous infections. If the PT does determine that an anatomical/biomechanical issue plays a leading role in a patient's pain, treating it can be a delicate balancing act. That's because more often than not, strengthening exercises and stretches are the treatment techniques involved. And by the time a person presents with pelvic pain, typically he/she has symptom-causing impairments, like trigger points or a too-tight pelvic floor, which may actually become exacerbated as a result of these techniques. So more often than not, the PT may have to first treat the symptom-causing impairment before turning his/her attention to the structural/biomechanical abnormality.

Skin Inspection

Several areas of the skin can give clues about the underlying causes of a patient's pelvic pain. Specifically, we look for these clues on the skin of the perineum, scrotum, and anus in men and the vulva, perineum, and anus in women. We're looking for any number of abnormalities that may correlate with a patient's symptoms. For instance, we're noting whether the skin is red, pale, discolored, blotchy, swollen, fissured, or looks abnormal in any way. Hemorrhoids are another issue we're checking for. This information can give us different clues to what's contributing to a patient's pain. For example, hemorrhoids and anal fissures mean the patient likely has chronic constipation and does a lot of straining, clueing us in that the patient's motor control will likely need to be addressed in PT. Another example is pale vulvar tissue that feels thin or lacks elasticity. This tells us that a patient might have hormonal issues contributing to her pain. In addition to looking at the skin and feeling for any abnormalities, we test for vulvar sensitivity in our female patients by using a test called the "Q-tip" test. Here we use a Q-tip to gently touch areas of the vulva. In an asymptomatic patient, the touch of a Q-tip would be benign. A patient with pelvic pain, however, might have as one of her symptoms irritated vulvar tissue. For this patient, the touch of a Q-tip might be extremely painful. If this is the case, it tells us that nerve, muscle, or tissue dysfunction might be contributing to the hypersensitivity of the patient's vulvar tissue. Lastly, in some patients, it might be relevant to check the reflexes associated with these areas for clues. For example, one reflex associated with the anus is the so-called "anal wink." Indeed, when touched, the anal sphincter is supposed to contract, causing the anus to wink similar to how an eye winks. Another reflex associated with the area involves the clitoris. When touched, the clitoris is supposed to move due to a contraction of the bulbospongiosus and ischiocavernosus muscles. If either of these reflexes is impaired, it might indicate something is occurring with the patient's sacral nerves (the nerves that supply the muscles and tissue responsible for urinary, bowel, and sexual function) and that further diagnostic tests are in order, such as an EMG, nerve conduction velocity test, MRI, or CT scan.

Internal Examination

The final step in the exam is the internal pelvic floor evaluation. Here we're looking for insight into the state of the pelvic floor muscles, pudendal nerve, and the connective tissue that surrounds the urethra in female patients and the prostate in male patients. With the exception of the bulbospongiosus in men, all these muscles can be accessed internally via the vagina or the anus (although some of the muscles, such as the obturator internus and the bulbospongiosus in women, can also be accessed externally). When evaluating the internal muscles of the pelvic floor, we must first assess the patient's overall pelvic floor motor control. When we refer to "motor control" of the pelvic floor, we're talking about whether a person has the ability to perform certain pelvic floor movements when asked. Specifically, we're assessing the ability to contract, relax, and lengthen the muscles. A lack of motor control indicates that the muscles are impaired. Regaining proper motor control is important because it will help improve pelvic floor muscle function and reduce symptoms. From there we assess each muscle of the pelvic floor for tightness, trigger points, and/or tenderness. This is done through gentle palpation. Next, we examine the internal nerves of the pelvic floor. This primarily involves all the branches of the pudendal nerve. When evaluating the pudendal nerve, we want to assess the tenderness of each branch. However, if we find that any of the nerve branches are irritated, we take special care not to further irritate them when treating the surrounding muscles. In addition, we'll work to figure out what, if any, other impairments or contributing factors are causing the irritation. For example, a tight obturator internus muscle might be causing nerve irritation. By treating this muscle we can create a healthy environment for the nerve, causing the nerve irritation to subside. Finally, we examine the connective tissue around the urethra and vulvar tissue in women and the connective tissue near the prostate in men. We're looking for restricted connective tissue.

IF . . . THEN CHECK FOR . . .

At the end of the day, the patient's symptoms lead us in our evaluation, whether we're working externally or internally. And indeed, although each pelvic pain case is different as far as impairments go, patterns do exist. Often it's as straightforward as: if the patient is feeling A, then the PT should seek to rule out B, C, or D. For example, if a woman complains of urethral burning, we'll know to check for impairments in the following areas, because those impairments are often the culprits with this symptom:

- the abdomen, inner/outer thighs, and bony pelvis for connective tissue dysfunction
- the abdominal muscles for trigger points
- the pelvic floor muscles, particularly the pubococcygeus and the periurethral connective tissue for tightness and poor mobility

- the pelvic floor muscles for motor control problems

Below we've compiled a cheat sheet of additional impairment patterns:

If . . . perineal pain in men . . . then check for . . .

- connective tissue dysfunction along the pelvis and in the abdomen and perineum,
- trigger points in the urogenital diaphragm (bulbospongiosus, ischioc-avernosus, transverse perineum), accessing the muscles both externally and internally when possible,
- and mobility of the perineal branch of the pudendal nerve.

If . . . pain with sitting . . . then check for . . .

- connective tissue dysfunction in the area of the pain, particularly the tissue around the sit bones, buttocks, and inner thighs and back of the thighs,
- trigger points and/or tightness in the pelvic floor muscles,
- trigger points (internally and externally) in the obturator internus muscle,
- and mobility of the perineal and/or rectal branch of the pudendal nerve.

If . . . pain upon vaginal penetration . . . then check for . . .

- trigger points or tightness in the urogenital diaphragm and adductors,
- connective tissue dysfunction in the vulvar tissue and the inner thighs,
- and mobility of the perineal and/or clitoral branch of the pudendal nerve.

If . . . pain post-ejaculation . . . then check for . . .

- connective tissue dysfunction in the inner thighs and lower abdomen,

- trigger points or tightness in the urogenital diaphragm,
- and mobility of the perineal and/or penile branch of the pudendal nerve.

If . . . tailbone pain . . . then check for . . .

- sacroiliac or sacrococcygeal joint dysfunction,
- trigger points or tightness in the iliococcygeus, pubococcygeus, and coccygeus muscles,
- connective tissue dysfunction in the buttocks, low back, and over the sacrum,
- trigger points in the obturator internus and piriformis muscles,
- and mobility of the inferior rectal branch of the pudendal nerve.

If . . . pain with bowel movements . . . then check for . . .

- trigger points or tightness in the puborectalis muscle and/or external anal sphincter,
- connective tissue dysfunction around the anus and in the buttocks,
- and mobility of the inferior rectal branch of the pudendal nerve.

If . . . urinary urgency/frequency . . . then check for . . .

- connective tissue dysfunction in the inner thighs and abdomen,
- trigger points and/or tightness in the pubococcygeus muscles,
- poor motor control of the pelvic floor muscles,
- and connective tissue dysfunction in the periurethral tissues.

MAKING A PLAN: MANAGING EXPECTATIONS AND SETTING GOALS

What we uncover during the patient evaluation gives us the information we need to start an effective treatment plan. An important part of embarking on a treatment plan with a patient is communicating expectations and goals. Toward that end, at the end of the first evaluation appointment, we give patients a clear idea of what we believe caused the onset of their symptoms, which identified impairments are causing their most bothersome symptoms, and how we're going to treat these impairments. In addition, we talk to the patient about what they can expect from PT, over the short term and over the long term. Obviously, a patient's ultimate goal with PT is to get better, but it's important to set more specific, attainable goals along the way, both long term and short term. For one thing, these goals give both PT and patient a benchmark to evaluate treatment progress. For another thing, setting *short-term* goals is one way to lay out reasonable expectations for the patient, and having reasonable expectations can play a major role in patient compliance and patience with the treatment process. For example, let's take the example of a female triathlete who has urinary urgency and frequency, pain with intercourse, vulvar itching, intolerance to pants, and inability to exercise without an increase in her bladder symptoms. Prior to coming to PT, her symptoms were present for three months following a series of urinary tract and yeast infections. Short-term goals (four to six PT visits) may be:

1. Patient will urinate no more than six to eight times in a 24-hour period.
2. Patient will be able to tolerate wearing loose pants.
3. Patient will not experience daily vulvar itching.

Layer by layer we address the impairments and reach goals. Every eight visits we note the patient's progress and reset the goals as well as the time frame surrounding them.

The set of goals for the next six to eight weeks might be:

1. Patient will be able to engage in intercourse without pain.
2. Patient will be able to run one mile without bladder symptoms.
3. Patient will be able to wear tight pants and jeans without discomfort.

Initially, we may see a patient one to two times per week for six to eight weeks. During this time we expect to see a change in their symptoms, as we are targeting the areas we believe play the largest role in their pain. Many patients reach their goals in three to six months of treatment, but some patients will need to be in treatment for longer, depending on the complexity of their case. Patients with more complex cases, meaning several different layers of contributing factors are involved in their pain, may take longer to reach their goals, like six months to one year. How long a patient has had pain, the severity of their symptoms, other medical issues happening concurrently, and whether a sensitized nervous system is a major component of their pain, all play a role in the rate at which patients improve.

MAKING A PLAN: AN INTERDISCIPLINARY APPROACH

In addition to setting goals with patients following their evaluation appointment, when necessary, we begin the process of making sure they have the right interdisciplinary treatment team in place. If they don't, we help them put one together. For example, if a patient already has providers on board who are helping them, we ask for their contact information so that we can send them our evaluation summary and call them if we have a question, need clarification on a component of their treatment plan, or want to discuss another treatment idea or strategy. Or if we believe a patient would benefit from interventions in addition to PT, we give them the necessary referrals. When suggesting additional treatment options for patients, like trigger point injections, Botox injections, or even medications, we always start with the most conservative treatments, meaning treatments that have the potential for maximum therapeutic benefit with the lowest risk. Once the patient has seen the referred provider or providers, we often get in contact with them to coordinate the best treatment strategy moving forward. Plus, it's always good to hear the other providers' impressions of the patient, so we can figure out if we need to change anything or add something to his/her treatment plan. As we've said before, when it comes to recovering from pelvic pain, working within an interdisciplinary treatment plan provides the greatest chance for our patients to meet their goals. Given that our role as providers is to tackle what is often one of the main drivers of a patient's symptoms and the fact that we'll see patients more frequently and for longer periods than other providers, we're more than willing to act as a facilitator of a patient's interdisciplinary plan.

WHERE THE CENTRAL NERVOUS SYSTEM FITS IN

Because we treat a persistent pain condition, we have to consider what role a sensitized nervous system plays in a patient's pain. Several clues can tip us off to whether a patient's sensitized central nervous system is behind his/her pain. For example, the patient may have a hard time describing the pain or where it's located. They may say something like, "It just kind of hurts all over." Another clue is if the patient's pain symptoms are spontaneous, meaning they seemingly occur without cause or an inciting activity. Lastly, the pain may be untrackable, meaning the patient can't really tell when it is going to flare up or why it happens. We begin uncovering what role the patient's central nervous system is playing in his/her pain during the initial evaluation interview. For example, a patient might tell us her pain started as pain with intercourse, then it evolved into constant vaginal pain, then the whole lower part of her body started to hurt, then she began having upper body pain, and now "everything" hurts. Now she can't even hold her partner's hand without increased vaginal pain, and any activity will increase it; six months ago, when her symptoms first started, she could still tolerate light exercise. When we're taking a patient's history, this kind of information indicates clearly that the nervous system is sensitized. In addition to altering the way we approach the patient's evaluation, if we determine a sensitized nervous system is heavily involved in a patient's pain, we work to figure out what other providers we can refer him/her to. Sometimes when patients hear that their pain might have a central nervous system component, they panic, wrongly believing it means nothing can be done for their symptoms. This couldn't be further from the truth! A number of treatment options are designed to treat a sensitized nervous system, from medication to acupuncture to a plethora of other techniques. (We provide more details about these in chapter 8.) While typically pain management doctors or psychologists have treated this issue, to date, a growing number of PTs are beginning to incorporate it into their therapy. Indeed, many pelvic floor PTs, us included, incorporate one particular technique into their treatment: pain education. To be sure, pain education has been proven to change the way patients perceive pain. In addition, it helps them overcome catastrophic thinking and fear avoidance behaviors, which in turn can alter their pain perception. At our clinics, we do a great deal of one-on-one pain physiology education with our patients during appointments. Not only do we ourselves discuss the information with them, we also refer them to a variety of well-vetted resources. Below is a list of a few of these resources:

- "Understanding Pain in Five Minutes," a video by the Body in Mind research team at the University of South Australia that's accessible at https://www.youtube.com/watch?v=4b8oB757DKc.
- "Why Things Hurt," a TED talk by neuroscientist Lorimer Moseley, Ph.D., of Samson Institute for Health Research at the University of South Australia, accessible at https://www.youtube.com/watch?v=gwd-wLdIHjs.
- *Explain Pain*, a book by David Butler, Australian physiotherapist and clinical researcher, and Lorimer Moseley (see appendix A).
- *Painful Yarns*, a book by Lorimer Moseley (see appendix A).
- *Understand Pain, Live Well Again* by Neil Pearson, which is available as a pamphlet as well as a PowerPoint presentation.

EVALUATION DAY: TAMRA'S STORY

Some might deem canceling a highly invasive surgery and deciding to fly out to San Francisco to see a PT recommended by online blog readers quite crazy. However, it turned out to be the best decision I ever made. I guess it makes sense to start at the beginning. I went to see Liz at PHRC because I had been suffering from unexplained vulvar and vaginal burning for several months. I immediately got a good feeling when I walked into the clinic because they had fancy cushions on their waiting room chairs. Imagine that—providing cushions for patients who have chronic pain problems! My appointment began with about 20 minutes of just talking about my medical history and previous symptoms. I basically filled Liz in on the past year and three months. In addition, she wanted to know my other medical history, like the fact that I was born with an inverted hip bone on my left side. After our talk she began the examination. The next hour she proceeded to do intense therapy on me. She began by doing external therapy, stimulating my muscles and connective tissue around the pelvic area. If you imagine the vagina as a triangle, she branched out on all three sides. "Massaging" isn't the proper word; it was harder than that. Liz called it "connective tissue manipulation" or "skin rolling." Certain parts were pretty painful, but tolerable. What is interesting is that I was in much more pain on the left side than the right. And indeed, Liz noticed my left side's muscles and tissue were much tighter. This point was further observed upon the inside examination and therapy. Her theory is that my left hip was never corrected when I was a child and may have initiated muscle imbalances, which my body compensated for so I could walk, but which have now evolved into pelvic floor dysfunction. The muscle imbalances cause my nerves to be hypersensitive, she said, and since a lot of nerves congregate around the pelvic floor, that's where I'm feeling the effects. The internal therapy hurt a lot in the beginning, but slowly I began to relax and not feel as much. Liz said she felt my muscles relax and respond to the treatment a few times, which is good news for my first PT appointment. The entire appointment took over two hours, and I learned a lot from Liz. She referred me to a PT in my city and she said she believed that with regular PT, in a year I would be fully recovered. To her, fully healed means "no cushion, bike riding, tampon using, sexually functioning, no pain ever again" recovered. Following my appointment, Liz e-mailed me an "evaluation summary," which listed all of her findings as well as her proposed treatment plan. I'm excited to pass this along to the PT I will see locally.

To wrap up, I just want to jot down some other points I took away from that first session:

- I've been wearing 100% cotton bikini underwear, but apparently the elastic is too tight for me. Elastic-less underwear will likely be less irritating.
- Liz said I would be sore a couple of days after therapy, especially externally. (She said it would feel like I had worked out really hard.) This was definitely true. It's been two days since therapy, and I'm still very sore. It seems to be worse along my two bikini lines and right below my top underwear line. But I like being sore, because I like feeling that progress is being made.
- PT is not a magic switch that's going to cure my pain in one day. Slowly my symptoms will begin to improve, and I will feel a decrease in pain levels.

A TYPICAL PELVIC PAIN PT TREATMENT SESSION

Now that we've covered the evaluation appointment, it's time to take a look at a typical pelvic pain PT session. At the beginning of a typical PT session, we walk into the room with the patient dressed and ask him/her pertinent questions to guide the treatment session. One important bit of information we want to get from patients is a description of their symptoms after their last treatment. We especially want to know how those first two or three days were after treatment. This is important for a few reasons. For one thing, oftentimes we'll focus our treatment for the day based on their response and what is bothering them the most. For another thing, it allows us to educate patients about reasonable expectations. For instance, if a patient is sore, we'll explain why that might be. (Soreness is common following PT, and while unpleasant, it is to be expected. Our patients often report that they feel "bruised.") On the other hand, an increase in their actual symptoms is obviously undesirable. When dealing with any pain syndrome, however, well-intended techniques can cause an increase in symptoms. These are typically transient and should resolve within 48 hours. If symptoms are better or worse after treatment, this tells us that we're targeting the right areas. Similar to the history, we want to know about the patient's most bothersome symptoms since the last appointment. For instance, if the patient has had pain with sex, we'll ask whether sex was possible. If it was, we'll want to know if anything was different about the experience. We'll want to know whether the pain was less in intensity, less in duration, or in a different area. A pelvic pain syndrome typically develops slowly over time, and the treatment process often follows suit. To be sure, a major symptom rarely goes away after one treatment. Rather, symptoms gradually become less bothersome after a series of treatments. And typically dysfunction changes before pain. For example, a patient with pudendal neuralgia may have burning perineal pain when sitting, and urinary hesitancy and frequency. The hesitancy and frequency may resolve completely as the burning pain with sitting declines over time. Clearly the burning pain is more bothersome, but the resolution of the urinary symptoms is a hint that things are improving. We typically spend the hour with a combination of manual therapy techniques, motor control exercises, and home program development. At the end of the appointment we review the overall game plan with the patient. For instance, we want them to know what changes to expect based on the techniques we used as well as the symptoms we expect to be unchanged based on what we didn't address. On the patient's end, their role is to comply with their home treatment program and lifestyle modifications we give them. And we encourage our patients to contact us immediately with any questions or concerns that come up between appointments.

MALE PELVIC PAIN: TREATING MEN RIGHT

As we've already made clear throughout the book, pelvic pain doesn't discriminate between the sexes. While it may be more prevalent in women for a variety of reasons—childbirth, vaginal infections, and hormonal fluctuations being the biggest—it is NOT a women's health issue! Men get it too. But when treating the condition, men with pelvic pain face their own set of challenges. For one thing, medical providers systematically misdiagnose any pelvic pain symptoms in men, including perineal pain, post-ejaculatory pain, urinary frequency, or penile pain, as a prostate infection, despite the absence of virus or bacteria. Typically the absence of a virus or bacteria simply means a switch in diagnosis from "prostate infection, or prostatitis" to "chronic nonbacterial prostatitis." And from there men are often prescribed antibiotics. In the beginning, because antibiotics have an analgesic effect, patients can actually feel a small improvement in symptoms. But before long, this effect wears off, and they're right back where they started. This situation exists despite the fact that in 1995, the National Institutes of Health (NIH) clearly stated that the diagnosis "chronic nonbacterial prostatitis" is incorrect for the symptoms of pelvic pain. To describe the symptoms, the NIH adopted the term "chronic pelvic pain syndrome." The symptoms the NIH listed for pelvic pain in men are painful urination, hesitancy, and frequency; penile, scrotal, anal, and perineal pain; and bowel and sexual dysfunction. On top of all that, despite the proven efficacy of PT for the treatment of pelvic pain, male patients as a whole have a harder time gaining access to a qualified pelvic floor PT. That's because not all pelvic floor PTs treat men. To date, the majority of pelvic floor PTs are women, and many female pelvic floor PTs are uncomfortable treating men. For some female PTs, it simply boils down to their not being comfortable dealing with the penis and scrotum. Among their qualms:

What if the patient gets an erection? How do I deal with that? Coming from a practice where about 30% of our patients are men with pelvic pain, here's our advice. If a male patient does get an erection, address it with a simple "Don't worry, it happens." And move on. But some female PTs are hesitant to treat male patients because they've received little to no training in treating the male pelvic floor. The good news is that in the past few years postgraduate-level classes (one of the main ways any PT receives education on pelvic floor rehabilitation) that focus on treating the male pelvic floor have become available for PTs, and more and more pelvic floor PTs are treating male patients. This is a big step in the right direction.

JUSTIN'S STORY

When I was 26, I woke up one day with urinary symptoms. Basically, I had a weak stream and felt as if I wasn't voiding completely. I also had a sensation in my urethra that's hard to describe. It wasn't pain, just a feeling of something being not quite right. Because the issue was urinary, I visited a urologist. The first doctor suspected either a prostate infection or a sexually transmitted disease. But all tests and cultures for either of those diagnoses came back negative. Nonetheless, the doctor diagnosed me as having "prostatitis," which is an infection of the prostate, and prescribed a course of antibiotics. When the medication didn't clear up my symptoms, I made an appointment with a second urologist, with the same outcome. In the course of a year, I saw about ten urologists, each of whom gave me a different course of antibiotics for "prostatitis" despite the fact that test after test came back negative for infection. After a year of urinary symptoms, the severity of which would wax and wane, I woke up one morning in the most pain I had ever been in in my life. It felt as if someone was stabbing me in the testicle with a knife. On top of that, I was having shooting pains in my anus and abdomen. The shooting pain was so severe, it literally sent me to my knees. I called two of the urologists I had the most faith in, and both said I was having "complications of prostatitis." At that point, I lost faith in these doctors' opinions as well as in the diagnosis of "prostatitis." Desperate for relief, I began searching online for answers. I focused my search on the prostate because I had never heard of pelvic pain, or the pelvic floor for that matter. In my search, I found an out-of-state doctor who was treating symptoms like mine by removing the prostate. Despite the possible side effects that come with that surgery—impotence, incontinence—I was in so much pain that I was seriously considering going that route. Eventually, the shooting pains disappeared, but I was left with constant testicular pain. Not knowing what was wrong was terrifying. Also, I had always been a very active person—very exercise conscious—but because of the pain and my fear of doing something to make it worse, I stopped working out completely. In fact, I stopped doing anything active and began to spend a lot of time either on the sofa or in bed. Thankfully, in the course of my research, I happened upon a pelvic pain online support group, and that's where I first learned about pelvic pain as well as pelvic floor PT. So I made an appointment with a PT on the East Coast, where I lived at the time, and began treatment. PT didn't help right away. Even though I was a super-compliant patient, it took about a year of regular PT and diligence with a home program for me to begin getting my life back. During that first year of PT, I lugged around a cushion everywhere I went for sitting and spent a lot of my time either on my sofa or in bed. I stopped drinking alcohol and caffeine, and I wasn't eating spicy foods because I was afraid all these things were contributing to my pain. And because of my pain and my anxiety surrounding it, I barely did anything social or that I enjoyed. My every waking moment became completely dictated by my pain. A big turning point came when I decided I needed to stop focusing on my symptoms and stop worrying that this would be something I would have for the rest of my life. That realization was life changing for me. That very week I went out with friends and had a couple of drinks, and thought, "Okay, I can have a normal life here." My mentality changed from that time forward. I found immediately that the less time I spent focusing on my pelvic pain, the better it got, and in turn the less I thought about it. I even began exercising again. I started swimming. It was an activity that allowed me to be active without flaring my symptoms. Then about a year into my pelvic pain, I moved to Los Angeles and began treatment with Stephanie at PHRC. By that time I was about 85% better, but I still had the testicular pain. It was improved, but was still there. What Stephanie found was that I lacked the motor control to relax my pelvic floor. Without the ability to do this, pelvic floor muscles will remain tight and become even tighter with exercise, thus continuing to produce pain. The first thing she taught me to do was relax my pelvic floor. Also, she found unresolved trigger points in several muscles that can cause testicular pain. So that's what we focused on in treatment. *So why did my symptoms start to begin with?* Stephanie's theory is that a combination of factors set off my pain. For one thing, I'm a super-active guy who's worked out hard with various trainers over the years. Add to that a history of low back pain, and voilà! Pelvic pain! After a few months of weekly PT with Stephanie, I am now pain-free. It was quite a journey! I learned a lot about myself along the way that I'll carry with me for the rest of my life. The benefits of relaxation and meditation are the most beneficial lesson I learned. I'm not really a spiritual person, but I now get how the mind-body connection works. I now have the tools to get stress out of my life, even if it's just for a few minutes a day. I know how to relax and be quiet, and I now understand that my mind has a huge impact on what happens with my body, and that I can work to control it. And another of the more interesting things that came out of my pelvic pain journey was learning just how common a problem it is. As soon as I began talking to others about what was happening with me, people I knew with pelvic pain issues or who knew someone who had pelvic pain issues began coming out of the woodwork, giving me a chance to share what I learned on my own journey. And basically that's number one: you need to see a qualified pelvic floor PT; and number two, recovery isn't going to be immediate, so you need to try your best to do whatever it takes to continue to live your life.

CONCLUSION

In this chapter, we've provided a look inside the PT treatment room. However, PT is but one treatment option available to those with pelvic pain. As we've already discussed in earlier chapters of the book, the most effective approach to treating pelvic pain is interdisciplinary, involving all appropriate providers. In the next chapter, we will discuss many of the treatment options offered by these other providers.

6

GUIDE TO NAVIGATING
TREATMENT OPTIONS

Besides PT, a variety of treatment options exist for pelvic pain. Having options is always a good thing, but often, deciding what treatments to try, and at what point during recovery, can be challenging. Due to the multilayered nature of pelvic pain, more often than not, the best approach to deciding between treatment options is a nuanced one that takes many factors into consideration—factors such as timing and whether certain treatments are best undertaken in combination with others. However, often these nuances are overlooked, and patients fall into a trap of either throwing everything but the kitchen sink at their pain—never a good approach because trying too many different treatments at once can be costly and lead to feelings of hopelessness and despair if symptoms persist—or giving up on certain treatments too soon because their expectations were off the mark. To help avoid these and other treatment pitfalls, we're devoting an entire chapter to how best to navigate the variety of different options now available to treat pelvic pain. We begin the chapter with a survey of the other treatment options, besides PT. From there, we'll explore what we consider to be the best strategy for navigating these different treatments. Finally, we'll end the chapter with a discussion on handling conflicting treatment advice from providers.

PELVIC PAIN TREATMENTS: A GUIDE

Dry Needling

Dry needling is a technique whereby fine needles are introduced into trigger points. The introduction of the needle into the trigger point "disrupts" the trigger point, helping to eradicate it. Medication is not used in conjunction with the placement of the needle. We consider this a safe and effective treatment option to eliminate trigger points. If this option is available to you, we suggest working it into your treatment plan, as most people with pelvic pain have problematic trigger points. Several different medical providers can perform dry needling, such as acupuncturists, physicians, nurse practitioners, physician assistants, and in most states, PTs.[1]

Injections

A few different injections exist to treat pelvic pain. The most common are trigger point injections, Botox injections, and nerve blocks. See the list below for a brief description of each.

- Trigger point injections: an anesthetic or anesthetic/steroid combination solution is injected into a trigger point. The theory behind the effectiveness of trigger point injections is that the introduction of the needle into the trigger point "deactivates" the trigger point, helping to eradicate it. The anesthetic used in the injection doesn't make the treatment more effective, it simply makes it more comfortable for the patient by numbing the area after the injection. A growing body of research supports the use of trigger point injections in the treatment of trigger points for pelvic pain. Physicians, physician assistants, and nurse practitioners can administer trigger point injections.[2]

When working to decide if trigger point injections are right for your treatment plan, you should ask your PT and/or physician the following questions:

1. *Which of my muscles have trigger points, and which of these, if any, do you think are contributing to my symptoms?* As we discussed in previous chapters, trigger points are a common impairment behind the symptoms of pelvic pain. However, just because a trigger point is present, doesn't mean it's relevant for a patient's most bothersome symptoms. Your provider can help you figure out if an identified trigger point is likely affecting your symptoms and if so, whether trigger point injections are an appropriate treatment approach.

2. *Do you think I should first try PT or dry needling to treat my trigger points before trying trigger point injections?* We always encourage patients to approach treatment using more conservative options first, and then to move to more invasive procedures if the conservative treatments are not effective. Typically, if we identify trigger points in our patients that do not respond to manual PT techniques in four to six appointments, that's when we recommend trigger point injections.

- Botox injections: botulinum toxin type A (Botox), a toxin produced by the bacterium *Clostridium botulinum*, is injected into a muscle with the aim of decreasing "muscle spasm," aka muscle contraction. Here's how: Botox acts as a nerve impulse "blocker," which prevents the release of chemical transmitters in charge of activating the muscle. By blocking these transmitters, the message to contract doesn't get to the muscle; therefore, the muscle doesn't spasm or contract. After about three months the medication is no longer active. Botox is a treatment option for too-tight pelvic floor muscles. It's typically used when muscles don't respond to conservative treatment, such as PT, or in cases where when coupled with PT, it can help hasten recovery. The jury is still out on possible long-term and short-term side effects of Botox injections for pelvic pain. When deciding if Botox injections are right for your treatment plan, we've compiled a list of questions worth considering.

  1. *Which of my muscles are "too tight," and which of these, if any, are contributing to my symptoms?* It's a good idea to ask your providers, either your PT or your physician, or both this question

to pinpoint if the muscles you're considering having Botoxed are indeed the muscles contributing to your symptoms.

2. *What are the risks of the injections?* In general, risks of Botox injections include urinary, gas, and fecal incontinence. This is especially the case when muscles around the urethral and anal sphincters are injected. When other muscles are injected, this potential side effect is not as much of a concern. A second potential side effect is that the muscles adjacent to the treated muscles may begin to compensate for the relaxation of their neighbors, causing new symptoms. Plus, there is the risk of the treatment causing an increase in pain.

3. *Is the therapeutic benefit worth the cost?* A limited number of providers offer Botox injections as a treatment for pelvic pain, necessitating travel. Also, most of the muscles injected for pelvic pain are not FDA approved; therefore, this procedure may not be covered by insurance. So when deciding whether to pursue Botox, patients often have to weigh financial factors into their decision.

4. *Am I going to have to keep getting these injections every three months to maintain the therapeutic benefits?* As mentioned above, the effects of Botox typically wear off after about three months. Typically, during that three-month window when the muscle/muscles are more relaxed, other treatments, such as PT, are administered, and the combination of treatments allows for expedited gains toward recovery. However, this is not always the case, and injections may need to be repeated in certain cases.

• Nerve blocks: medication is injected around a specific nerve for various purposes. These injections can contain an anesthetic (numbing medication) only or an anesthetic combined with a steroid (anti-inflammatory medication). In the context of treating pelvic pain, nerve blocks are typically used for three different purposes:

• as a therapeutic treatment to try to control acute nerve pain,
• as a diagnostic tool to try to determine the source of a particular symptom,
• or as a prognostic indicator to determine if a more permanent treatment (such as surgery) would be successful in treating symptoms.

If you have nerve-like pain (burning, stabbing, shooting) in a particular distribution of a specific nerve branch, a nerve block may be appropriate.

However, within the pelvic pain provider community, a wide array of opinions exist surrounding the effectiveness of nerve blocks as well as when and how they should be administered. For example, different opinions exist as to exactly what medications should be used in the blocks. And very little research is available to clear up these questions. So when deciding whether a nerve block is right for you, we recommend you ask the provider recommending the treatment exactly what he/she expects to achieve with the block. Specific questions to ask include:

- What is the exact purpose of the block? Is it to decrease symptoms or for diagnostic purposes?
- What are the potential side effects of the injection? Is it possible that it may increase my symptoms?
- If the purpose of the block is to lessen symptoms, to what degree and how long with the relief last?

Topical Options

A variety of topical medications are commonly prescribed for people dealing with pelvic pain. The majority of these medications are prescribed to female patients, as they are targeted to vulvar or vaginal tissue. One of the more common of these medications is topical estrogen, which is prescribed when estrogen levels are not at optimal levels, causing problems for a woman's vulvar tissue or vagina. Another common topical medication used to treat pelvic pain, particularly in women, is lidocaine. Lidocaine is an anesthetic, or numbing agent, which in ointment or cream form can be applied to areas of hypersensitivity or pain. For example, women with vulvar pain can apply it to the areas of their vulva that are painful or hypersensitive, enabling them to wear underwear or jeans with less discomfort. Some women with pelvic pain use it in place of, or in addition to, lubrication during intercourse to decrease the pain or hypersensitivity they feel during penetration. Other topical medications used to treat pelvic pain are compounded medications. A compounded medication includes several medications mixed together in one ointment or cream that can then be applied to the skin and/or vulvar tissue. These compounded medications can combine an anesthetic, like lidocaine; an anticonvulsant, like gabapentin; a muscle relaxer, like baclofen; a tricyclic, like amitriptyline; and/or a pain medication, like ketamine. However, these medications are not commonly prescribed by the average gynecologist or primary care physician, so seeking a consult with a pelvic pain specialist may be the best course of action if you want to try a compounded medication. Currently, research does not exist as to the efficacy of these compounded medications for treating pelvic pain symptoms.

Medications

Four categories of medications are commonly used to treat the various symptoms of pelvic pain. They are:

- neuropathic analgesics,
- anticonvulsants,
- N-methyl-D-aspartate (NMDA) antagonists,
- and benzodiazepines.

Neuropathic analgesics are antidepressant medications used to treat neuropathic pain. Examples are tricyclics and mixed reuptake inhibitors, or SNRIs. Tricyclic antidepressants are widely used for treating pelvic pain. Amitriptyline is the most commonly studied and has been shown to be an effective treatment for neuropathic pain.[3] Anticonvulsants have been used in pain management for many years. The two most common examples used to treat persistent pain are gabapentin (Neurontin) and pregabalin (Lyrica). Gabapentin has been reported to be well tolerated and an effective treatment in various pain conditions, particularly in neuropathic pain.[4] NMDA antagonists have also been useful in treating persistent pain conditions.[5] Ketamine is one example of this group of medications. Benzodiazepines are often used for treating symptoms such as anxiety, sleep difficulties, and muscle spasm. A commonly prescribed benzodiazepine is diazepam, or Valium. This medication can be taken orally, or as many people with pelvic pain take it, by vaginal or rectal suppository. In fact, several of the above-mentioned medications, such as neurontin and amitriptyline, can also be administered in suppository form either individually or as a compounded combination. A word about opiates to treat pelvic pain: according to the National Guideline Clearinghouse, a public resource for evidence-based clinical practice guidelines, the role of opiates for the treatment of pelvic pain is limited, and they should only be started in consultation with all parties involved (including the patient's family practitioner). National guidelines exist and should be followed. There is a growing understanding of the limitations of opioid use, and more recently, the paradoxical situation of opioid-induced hyperalgesia. Recent research shows that the above-mentioned classes of medications are more effective and safer for patients with nonmalignant pain.[6]

It's important for patients and their team to work together to figure out if and when certain medications are appropriate. In certain cases, the side effects or cost may outweigh the therapeutic benefit. What's more, although the medications discussed above have strong research to support their effectiveness for treating pain, exactly what this means will vary widely from patient to patient. For one patient, a certain medication will greatly impact his/her symptoms, but for another it may simply allow him/her to tolerate other treatments or prevent his/her nervous system from becoming more sensitized than it already is. Another important consideration is the therapeutic dose of the medication and the length of time needed to achieve that dose. For instance, it's possible that a medication appeared ineffective to a patient because he/she wasn't on a high enough dose and/or took the medication for too short a period of time, not giving it a chance to "kick in."

Neuromodulation

Neuromodulation is a technology that acts directly on nerves by altering or modulating their activity, delivering electrical stimulation to specific nerve distributions. The three kinds of neuromodulation most commonly used for the treatment of pelvic pain are tibial nerve stimulation, sacral neuromodulation, and pudendal nerve stimulation. Tibial nerve stimulation is done weekly on an outpatient basis for 12 weeks. It has been primarily used for urinary dysfunction, but emerging research suggests it may be a safe, minimally invasive, and inexpensive treatment option for pelvic pain.[7] While minimally invasive, tibial nerve stimulation is limited by patients needing to make weekly visits for treatment.

Sacral neuromodulation has been used successfully for many years for urinary dysfunction, and again, some promising research has supported its use for pelvic pain, but the jury is definitely still out on its effectiveness.[8]

Sacral neuromodulation is performed by implanting an electrical stimulating device on the third sacral nerve root, which carries information, including pain, to the brain. Pudendal nerve stimulation is a newer form of neuromodulation currently being studied and used experimentally. Instead of implanting the stimulating device onto the sacral nerve, the device is placed directly on the pudendal nerve, which also carries pain information from the pelvis to the brain. No determined protocol states when a person should consider neuromodulation. In most cases of both sacral and pudendal neuromodulation, a one-week trial is performed where the stimulator remains on the skin, but the patient can still determine if it causes pain relief. If relief is obtained, the device gets surgically implanted onto the nerve or nerve root. These procedures are often covered by insurance and may be worth considering if a patient's pain is not responding to more conservative treatments.

Continuous or Pulsed Radiofrequency

Continuous and pulsed radiofrequency use current to destroy tissue that carries pain signals. With continuous radiofrequency the current is applied continuously during treatment, whereas with pulsed radiofrequency it's applied using brief "pulses." The current is applied to the nerve itself through the skin via a needle. The theory is that eliminating fibers that cause pain will reduce symptoms for patients. Recent literature has shown that pulsed radiofrequency is safer than continuous radiofrequency.[9] However, to date, research regarding whether it's an effective treatment for pelvic pain is lacking.

Surgical Treatment Options

As we've discussed throughout this book, conservative treatment for pelvic pain is always the first and most desirable treatment approach. However, surgical intervention is necessary in some situations. As we've already discussed, many different contributing factors can be involved in pelvic pain. At times surgery is needed to treat a specific contributing factor. For example, surgery may be necessary to treat an underlying gynecological condition or an orthopedic issue. Because so many different surgeries are associated with the factors that can contribute to pelvic pain, it's impossible for us to cover all of them in this book; however, we would like to review a handful of the more commonly performed surgical procedures associated with pelvic pain, including pudendal nerve decompression surgery, a vestibulectomy, a laparoscopy, and surgical mesh removal. Below is a brief description of each.

Pudendal nerve decompression surgery

When the pudendal nerve becomes compressed or "entrapped," the condition is referred to as pudendal nerve entrapment or PNE, and the surgery used to release the nerve is called pudendal nerve decompression surgery. Symptoms of PNE are typically the same as symptoms of pudendal neuralgia and include stabbing, shooting, or burning pain anywhere along the trajectory of the pudendal nerve. The pudendal nerve can become entrapped in a variety of different ways; for example, as the result of surgery, such as when mesh is used to correct a prolapse, or as a result of scar tissue formation, such as from childbirth or a fall to the buttock area. Because there is no way to definitively diagnose PNE, it's a diagnosis of exclusion. In making the diagnosis, consideration of a patient's history is key. And the main indicator as to whether he/she has an entrapped nerve is whether a traumatic event or events have taken place. Besides the patient history, surgeons use several diagnostic tests to help them determine, along with a patient history and evaluation, whether someone is a good candidate for surgery. However, at the end of the day, it's impossible for a physician to say with 100% certainty that a nerve is entrapped. And even when entrapment is suspected, often patients are initially steered toward more conservative treatments, such as Botox injections, nerve blocks, medication to reduce nerve hypersensitivity, PT, and lifestyle changes, such as limiting sitting or other physical activities that increase pain. If those treatments are unsuccessful and a patient opts for surgery, there is no guarantee that it will be successful. If a patient does go the surgery route, he/she will likely need to continue to pursue other treatments as well. In fact, the biggest impact of the surgery may be that it allows other treatments, like nerve blocks or PT, to be more successful by decreasing nerve irritation. For more detailed information about pudendal nerve decompression surgery, check out a Q&A on our blog with the two top surgeons who perform the operation in the United States: Dr. Mark Conway, attending gynecologist and pelvic surgeon at St. Joseph's Hospital in Nashua, New Hampshire; and Dr. Michael Hibner, the director of the Arizona Center for Chronic Pelvic Pain at St. Joseph's Hospital and Medical Center in Phoenix. (See http://www.pelvicpainrehab.com/pelvic-pain/1893/pne-your-questions-answered/ and http://www.pelvicpainrehab.com/pelvic-pain/1901/pne-your-questions-answered-part-ii/.)

Vestibulectomy

This is a surgical procedure indicated for certain women with localized provoked vestibulodynia (pain in the vestibule when touched or provoked) when more conservative treatment measures have failed. During the procedure, the surgeon removes the painful tissue. As with many of the surgical treatment options for pelvic pain, this procedure is rife with controversy within the medical community. What is most important in opting for this surgical treatment is determining whether or not you're an appropriate candidate. For the most part, that means that the patient's pain is coming from the inflamed vestibular tissue only and not from other contributing factors. Indeed, research has shown that for the right candidate, a vestibulectomy can be effective.[10] If you're a woman with provoked vestibulodynia and have failed conservative treatment, you may benefit from consulting with a pelvic pain specialist to determine if you are a good candidate for this treatment option.

Laparoscopy

Laparoscopy is a surgical procedure that uses a thin, lighted tube inserted through the belly to view or remove abdominal organs and/or female pelvic organs. The procedure is performed for many pelvic-pain-related reasons, such as removing organs like the uterus, removing abnormal growths like tumors or fibroids, or removing unwanted or pathological tissue like endometriosis. A decision on laparoscopy as a treatment option for a persistent pelvic-pain-related contributing factor needs to be carefully made under the guidance of a pelvic pain specialist.

Surgical mesh removal

Surgical mesh is a synthetic material that is commonly used in the surgical repair of hernias and some pelvic floor disorders. Mesh has received a lot of attention in the media lately for postsurgical complications associated with its use. Some of those complications can cause pelvic pain and therefore, a surgical procedure may be warranted to remove all or part of the mesh. One recent study examined the effects on pelvic pain after mesh revision or removal, and 73% of women reported an improvement in pain, 8% that their pain increased, and 19% reported that their pain was unchanged.[11] If you developed pelvic pain after a surgical procedure that involved mesh, we strongly encourage you to seek a consultation with a pelvic pain specialist to discuss your treatment options.

TREATING A SENSITIZED NERVOUS SYSTEM

In the past, when it was determined that a sensitized nervous system played a role in a patient's pain, the main line of treatment was medication. Fast-forward to today. While medication remains a viable option, these days a slew of other treatments are available to dial down a sensitized nervous system. These treatments are predicated on the fact that many cognitive processes play a role in how we perceive pain—processes like thoughts, emotions, and beliefs. So anxiety, stress, catastrophic thinking, fear avoidance—all these emotions/patterns of thinking—can impact how we perceive pain. Now that's not to say your pain is all in your head, and if you'll only "stop stressing and relax," it'll go away. If only it were that simple! No, what we're saying is that the brain is 100% responsible for how we perceive pain, and other things that go on in the brain—thoughts, emotions, beliefs—can impact that perception. By working to alter these cognitive processes, you can dial down a sensitized nervous system, and thus your pain. That's not to say it's an easy undertaking or it's a process that works overnight. Turning down the volume on a sensitized nervous system often takes time and commitment. And you don't have to figure it out on your own. Many patients turn to a psychologist to help them put a plan together. Plus, as we mentioned in the previous chapter, pelvic floor PTs can also play a role in the process, namely by educating patients on the physiology of their pain in order to remove some of the anxiety and fear surrounding it. In addition, they can identify certain thought patterns and behaviors, like catastrophic thinking or fear avoidance, and both address them with the patient and refer him/her to a psychologist or other appropriate provider. Below are some techniques commonly used to treat a sensitized nervous system. (Note: it's far from a definitive list!)

- Changing thought patterns, such as catastrophic thinking or fear avoidance around certain activities
- Relaxation training: these techniques are aimed at calming down the nervous system on a body-wide level with activities such as meditation, tai chi, yoga, deep breathing techniques, acupuncture, massage, and hypnosis.
- Guided imagery: this technique is designed more toward targeting the exact location of a patient's symptoms. Guided imagery directs thoughts and suggestions toward a relaxed and focused state. While a provider can walk you through guided imagery, you can also use tapes or a script. For instance, a DVD called *Guided Imagery for Women with Pelvic Pain, Interstitial Cystitis or Vulvodynia* is available for pelvic pain patients. For more information on this DVD, go to http://www.healthjourneys.com/Store/Products/Guided-Imagery-for-Women-with-Pelvic-Pain-Interstitial-Cystitis-or-Vulvodynia/527.
- Addressing sleep dysfunction: not getting enough rest is detrimental to a sensitized nervous system, so getting a good night's sleep regularly is a must.

COGNITIVE BEHAVIORAL THERAPY

Cognitive behavioral therapy (CBT) is a form of psychotherapy designed to treat problems by changing negative thinking, emotions, and thoughts. Those dealing with pelvic pain can often benefit from CBT. For one thing, it can help change their emotional responses to pain as well as any negative behavior patterns surrounding their pain. The desired outcome of CBT is to reduce distress for the patient while improving daily functioning by arming them with tools for coping and problem solving. Many of the treatment strategies used in CBT overlap with those for treating a sensitized nervous system. The main differentiator is that the goal with CBT is to improve a patient's outlook and daily functioning, while treating a sensitized nervous system is about changing how his/her brain is processing pain. However, ultimately, achieving the goals of the former will help toward achieving the goals of the latter.

Reprogramming My Sensitized Nervous System: Olivia's Story

My pain began after a routine gynecological surgery, which was followed by an undiagnosed vaginal bacterial infection that lasted for several months. My main symptoms were sit bone pain and pain down the back of my leg, plus an awful, prickly vulvar pain. About a year and a half into my symptoms, I traveled out-of-state to visit Stephanie, who found trigger points in my hip muscles and one in my right bulbospongiosus muscle, severe connective tissue restriction on my thighs and vulvar tissue, as well as some nerve irritation of my posterior femoral cutaneous nerve. When I got back home, I continued PT with a local therapist. In addition, I saw a chiropractor and used a topical nerve cream on my vulvar tissue and the back of my legs. As a result of these treatments, my sit bone pain and the pain down the back of my legs resolved. However, the awful prickly sensation I felt on my vulva persisted. I was two years into this pain, and it was really preventing me from living a normal life. Discouraged and frustrated, I began to research the central nervous system, chronic pain, and anxiety. I also started to see a health psychologist. (Health psychology is a specialty that focuses on how biological, social, and psychological factors influence health and illness.) My health psychologist confirmed what I was starting to figure out on my own. My fear of my symptoms was continuing my pain cycle, and in order to fully recover, I'd have to work to heal my nervous system. This was a huge breakthrough for me. But I knew it wasn't going to be easy. The first thing I did was take a break from PT and the chiropractor so that I could focus on my mental and emotional well-being. I knew I could always return to either at any time. My biggest problems from an emotional standpoint were that I had tremendous anxiety and hypervigilance around my symptoms. Even though I was feeling better and my day-to-day life had improved, I simply couldn't stop thinking about my pain. It was always in the back of my mind, affecting everything I did. The first thing I did to overcome this was to pick up a copy of a book titled *Hope and Help for Your Nerves* by Claire Weekes. The book helped me understand the nervous system and how to heal it. With the help of my therapist and the book, I began working to allow my symptoms to just be, without the tension and fear I invariably heaped on top of them. I had come to realize that this tension and fear was continuing my pain cycle by keeping my nervous system aroused. I also started wearing underwear, a pain trigger for me, every day, even if it was just for an hour. I needed my mind and body to remember that underwear was not a threat. Although it took several weeks, ultimately, wearing underwear began to feel normal again. I took the same approach to sitting. When I would have symptoms with sitting, I'd say to myself, "I feel this or that, and that's okay because there is no injury. It's just my nervous system." I also worked to keep myself busy and not focus on my pain while going about my day. Plus, I gave myself breaks to just relax. I even allowed myself at least one nap a day to make sure I was getting enough rest. After a few months, my plan began to pay off. I had about a two-and-a-half-month stretch of no pain! Encouraged, I began working out again. When I would notice symptoms as a result of my workout, I might back off a little, but I continued the activity. I knew I needed to expose myself to these situations to allow my nervous system to heal. Life became a lot easier, but for some reason, I still felt depressed, sad, and exhausted. The depression worsened, causing my nervous system to become worked up again. My prickly vulvar symptoms returned. I was so disappointed. After visiting my doctor for some blood work, it was uncovered that I had an overactive thyroid. Within two weeks of taking medication for the problem, I noticed an improvement in my mood. Eventually I began feeling well enough emotionally to once again begin allowing my symptoms to exist without reacting. Within a couple of months, I was again symptom-free. I'm fully aware that symptoms can return at any time, but if they do, I'll do my best to have less of a reaction to them and not get my nervous system aroused. I have tools in my toolbox now. I view my recovery as a remission. This remission could go on forever, or I could have a flare-up. The important thing for me to remember is if I do have a flare-up, my symptoms will go away.

DIAGNOSTIC TESTING

A slew of diagnostic tests can come into play when it comes to pelvic pain, such as bladder cystoscopy, vulvar biopsy, colonoscopy/endoscopy for IBS, or 3-Tesla MRI of the pelvis, to name a few. Certain diagnostic tests run the risk of causing pain flares and/or may be expensive, involving time and travel. Therefore, we advise patients to ask their providers exactly how the outcome of the test will change their treatment plan. Oftentimes the answer is that although it might give certain nuanced information to the provider, it may not have an impact on the patient's overall treatment plan. If the end result is not going to change and/or improve the patient's treatment plan, a particular test may not be the best use of patients' resources.

ALTERNATIVE MEDICINE

In addition to traditional Western medicine, certain alternative treatments can offer therapeutic benefit to those recovering from pelvic pain with relatively low risk. If our patients are having success with an alternative practitioner, we always encourage them to continue with that practitioner. And when referring patients to an alternative practitioner, as with any referral we give patients, we only refer to practitioners whom we've had experience with or whom we know well enough to feel confident that their services will benefit the patient. And we prefer to refer to practitioners who have some experience with and/or knowledge of pelvic pain. When we do refer patients to an alternative medicine practitioner, we do so for very specific services. Examples include:

- A naturopathic doctor may be beneficial for women who are struggling with chronic vaginal infections that have failed traditional treatment protocols or for patients who need help regulating their gastrointestinal, urinary, and vaginal balance to eliminate or prevent infections or to reduce symptoms of irritable bowel syndrome.
- A medical hypnosis practitioner may be helpful for a patient with a sensitized nervous system, or who is struggling with anxiety and is not interested in medication.

- An acupuncturist can administer dry needling for trigger points. Acupuncture may also help reduce overall pain and nervous system hypersensitivity and regulate sleep.

Alternative therapies can get costly, so we always advise patients to be very clear about what their goals and expectations are for treatment. A goal of "alleviating pain" is too broad. A more specific goal, such as "I'm hoping a naturopath can help me overcome my constipation so that I can eliminate it as a contributing factor to my pelvic pain," is much more on target. Having specific goals in place helps patients figure out if the treatments are helping and are worth continuing.

PUTTING IT ALL TOGETHER

Part of taking on the role of treatment facilitators for our patients is providing them with information and guidance when figuring out their interdisciplinary treatment approach. In doing so, we always suggest a "highest benefit with lowest risk" approach to choosing between different treatment options, meaning we counsel patients to first try more conservative treatments, such as PT, dry needling, or medication, before treatments that carry higher risk, such as Botox injections, nerve blocks, or surgery. Another consideration is timing. Oftentimes one layer of a patient's pain must be cleared up before another is targeted, such as a case where a patient's central nervous system must first be dialed down in order for manual PT techniques to be tolerated or effective. Plus, certain treatments work best in combination with others. For example, Botox or trigger point injections often work well in combination with PT and medication. Lastly, treatment for pelvic pain is a dynamic process that involves constant assessment and reassessment by all providers involved in a patient's treatment team. Regular reevaluations and discussions help a patient's treatment team determine the effects of current and past treatments as well as which therapeutic strategies to implement next as the patient improves.

HANDLING CONFLICTING INFORMATION FROM PROVIDERS

As we've already discussed throughout this book, when it comes to treating pelvic pain, an interdisciplinary approach is the way to go. However, at times patients may receive conflicting information from providers. Given the nature of pelvic pain—the fact that several contributing factors and impairments are often involved, requiring providers from across medical specialties to weigh in—differences of opinion among providers are bound to happen. Plus, even the best of medical specialists can get tripped up by a complex pelvic pain case and won't always know the best treatment approach to take. Lastly, it's worth bearing in mind that medical providers aren't always immune to the truth behind the saying "If all you have is a hammer, everything looks like a nail." But we understand how intimidating and challenging it can be for patients when their providers don't agree. Too often we have patients come to us with multiple diagnoses from multiple providers, for example. In fact, chances are if you're a female reader with pelvic pain, you've likely been diagnosed by a gynecologist with vulvodynia, by a urologist with interstitial cystitis, and by a gastroenterologist with IBS. Getting multiple diagnoses from physicians understandably leads to confusion and frustration. In addition, providers will on occasion offer conflicting opinions on treatment options. One fairly common example is when one provider recommends a nerve block while another tells the patient he/she should absolutely not get a nerve block. In such a scenario, it's best to ask each provider what his/her reasons are for their recommendations. Other questions to ask include: What is the desired effect of the treatment? What are the possible negative side effects? Are there alternative treatments to achieve the same goal? Once patients have all the information from each of their providers, they can then make a more informed decision. Another thing to keep in mind is that as we've discussed previously, not many providers have a lot of experience treating pelvic pain conditions. So if you get conflicting medical advice regarding your pelvic pain, consider your provider's experience treating pelvic pain specifically. He/she may be the world-renowned expert in another subset of medicine but have very little experience treating pelvic pain. And the specialists who treat pelvic pain will each have specific tests and treatments that they recommend and administer to patients. This is yet another reason we encourage patients to have one provider "driving" their care. This provider can help them sort through any different opinions they get from other members of their team. It is our philosophy, and we hope others adopt it, that if we cannot help our patient, we will help them get to the person or people that can.

In this chapter, we've provided a survey of the many treatment options available to treat pelvic pain. As the information above makes clear, no road map exists for putting together an appropriate treatment plan for a pelvic pain syndrome. Rather it's an exercise best approached with thoughtfulness and care and in consultation with your treatment team. Our hope is that the guidance we've presented above will help both patients and providers tackle the task.

7

THE PELVIC FLOOR AND PREGNANCY: TREATING NEW MOMS RIGHT

After her first pregnancy, Angela gave birth to a beautiful 7-pound, 3-ounce baby girl. More than six months after leaving the hospital, baby was healthy and thriving; however, the same couldn't be said for mom. Mentally, despite the sleep deprivation, she was full of joy over being a new mom, but physically . . . well, physically, she just didn't feel right. For one thing, every time she laughed or coughed, she leaked urine. And when she went for her first run after giving birth, she leaked and could not control gas. Before attempting the run, at her six-week postpartum follow-up appointment, she had told her ob-gyn about the leaking issue. Her doctor reassured her that a little leaking was normal after childbirth and instructed her to do Kegels. Then he cleared her for resuming sex and exercise, which brings us to the other reason Angela "wasn't feeling quite right." Before the baby, she and her husband had had a healthy sex life; now, post-baby, for Angela sex was painful. Anytime she and her husband would attempt intercourse, she would feel pain upon penetration. After a few more reassurances from her doctor that everything was fine, Angela figured that she'd better start getting used to her "new normal": painful sex, no more running, and occasional incontinence. *Oh well, I guess it's all part of having kids,* she thought. Angela is one of millions of new moms who believe that postpartum pelvic floor symptoms are all part of a new normal that they "just have to get used to." But Angela's symptoms and the host of other symptoms new moms can face after pregnancy and delivery, or during pregnancy for that matter, are far from "normal." In fact, the vast majority of common pregnancy and postpartum pelvic floor issues *are* treatable.

In this chapter we're going to take a close look at common pregnancy and postpartum pelvic floor issues that cause both pain and dysfunction. We'll begin the chapter with a discussion of the pelvic floor–related problems that can arise during pregnancy. Then we'll take a look at the problems that crop up after the baby is born. We'll end the chapter with a discussion of two common pregnancy/postpartum concerns we've heard time and again from new moms over the years: returning to exercise post-baby and navigating pregnancy if you're a woman with a history of pelvic pain.

PELVIC FLOOR PROBLEMS DURING PREGNANCY

Countless physical changes come with pregnancy, and not surprisingly many of those changes impact the pelvic floor. For one thing, pregnancy puts additional pressure on the muscles of the pelvic floor because of the added weight that inevitably comes along with it. So the pelvic floor muscles have to work even harder to hold/support everything in the abdomen as well as maintain continence. The pelvic floor muscles are designed for this amped-up role during pregnancy, however, so typically they'll bounce back to normal postpartum (but not always; more on this in the section below). But there are times when the muscles become so overtaxed during pregnancy that problems arise, such as urinary incontinence. Problems can also arise as a result of the postural changes that occur during pregnancy. Typically pregnancy causes a significant change in posture. Indeed, as the mom-to-be's abdomen and breasts become larger, her center of gravity is pushed forward, her low back becomes curved, her upper back becomes rounded, and her head is pushed forward to compensate for the new weight distribution. Hormonal changes during pregnancy are also behind pelvic floor–related problems. For example, a hormone called relaxin is released during pregnancy to soften and ultimately open the pelvic joints in preparation for delivery. This change can result in a feeling of instability as well as contribute to back pain and a loss of balance.

Below we've compiled a list of some of the more common problems that can crop up during pregnancy.

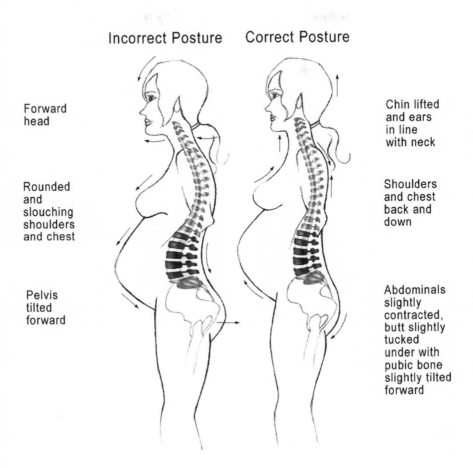

Figure 7.1. Comparison of incorrect and correct posture during pregnancy.
Source: Pelvic Health and Rehabilitation Center

- Foot and back pain, specifically low back pain
- Neck pain and headaches due to changes in posture
- Sciatic, hip, sacral, pelvic girdle, and tailbone pain
- Urine leakage due to pelvic floor muscle dysfunction
- Round ligament pain: the round ligament supports the uterus as it grows

Women often talk to their ob-gyns about musculoskeletal pain during pregnancy. However, often they don't get referred to PT. The thinking is that their pain is caused by their pregnancy, which is only going to advance, so "why bother?" But while these problems are "common," they are not "normal," and a pregnant woman should not be left to power through the pain and discomfort she feels when solutions are available for help and relief. But the reality is that ob-gyns are not going to focus on a pregnant patient's musculoskeletal issues, so it may be best for an expectant mom to look to her primary care physician for counsel when she encounters any of the above-mentioned issues and to ask for a PT referral. Indeed, a pelvic floor PT can help with all the above-mentioned symptoms in part with manual therapy and therapeutic exercises aimed at decreasing pain, but also by educating patients on certain lifestyle modifications that can further help to decrease pain/discomfort/dysfunction. For example, a PT can make recommendations for more supportive footwear or shoe inserts or offer advice on how to support the low back and/or sacroiliac joint if there is instability. Plus, she can school expectant moms about shoulder- and neck-friendly ways to hold the baby during breastfeeding as well as back-friendly methods to hoist their new bundles of joy from the crib, floor, or stroller. More good news: in addition to treating pregnancy-related pain or discomfort, a pelvic floor PT can also deploy techniques that can actually better position a woman physically for delivery. For instance, a PT can work with an expectant mom to improve her pelvic floor motor control (improving motor control simply means to improve the strength, endurance, and ability to relax the pelvic floor muscles), which in turn will help her push more effectively during labor. Becoming a whiz at controlling your pelvic floor won't just help with pushing; it also has the potential to save you from encountering problems postpartum, such as leaking urine when laughing, sneezing, coughing, or exercising. A PT can further help prepare the pelvic floor muscles for a smooth delivery by assessing the muscles to make sure they're in the best possible shape. The pelvic floor muscles and core stabilizing muscles are intimately involved in the childbirth process. These muscles function at their maximum potential when they're lengthened, strengthened, and free of trigger points. Impaired muscles are not always symptomatic, so a mom-to-be can have a problem and not even realize it, a problem that has the potential to set her up for postpartum issues. A PT can examine each muscle individually, both internally and externally. If impairments are found, they can be treated with manual therapy and exercise. Lastly, a PT can teach an expectant mom techniques that may help prevent or lessen the degree of perineal tearing. (The perineum is the area of skin between the vagina and the anus.) This technique is called perineal massage, the practice of massaging a pregnant woman's perineum in preparation for childbirth. Typically the PT teaches both the mom-to-be and her partner this technique. The theory behind perineal massage is that massaging the tissue increases muscle and tissue elasticity, thus decreasing the likelihood of the perineum tearing (or if it does tear, decreasing the severity of the tear) during birth or during an instrument (forceps or vacuum extraction) delivery. In addition, the technique is aimed at lowering the need for an episiotomy.[1]

PELVIC GIRDLE PAIN

One of the more common pelvic pain–causing conditions that occurs during pregnancy is called pelvic girdle pain or PGP. PGP happens when pregnancy hormones cause the tendons and ligaments that secure and stabilize the pelvis to become more lax, leaving the bones suscepti-ble to slipping out of place. The pelvis is made up of two bones joined to the base of the spine in two places, and then at the front to the pubic bone. It's designed to be strong enough to support the body but flexible enough to absorb the impact of the feet hitting the ground. PGP occurs when the bones become misaligned at the pelvic joints. Sometimes the joints can even lock up, leaving the woman temporarily unable to move one or both legs. According to research, PGP occurs in 50% of pregnant women.[2] Despite the high occurrence of the condition and the fact that it's treatable, more often than not, women either get no treatment at all or the wrong treatment, leaving them with pain in the back, leg, hip, buttock, and/or at the front of the pelvis as well as making them vulner-able to PGP during future pregnancies. The pain can be debilitating. Proper pelvic floor PT is the best treatment for PGP because it enables a woman to become more functional and experience less pain during the course of her pregnancy as well as during her labor and delivery. Here is a comprehensive list of all the strategies used by pelvic floor PTs to treat PGP:

- manual therapy techniques for soft tissue problems and joint dys-function,

- stabilization exercises,
- stabilization tools such as orthotics and sacroiliac joint belts,
- and patient education for lifestyle and biomechanical modifications.

AFTER THE BABY: COMMON POSTPARTUM PELVIC FLOOR PROBLEMS

The pelvic floor takes a real beating during even a "normal" childbirth. Here's a play-by-play of exactly what happens to the pelvic floor during delivery: The skin layers of the vagina will stretch often to the point of tearing, requiring stitches. Also the pelvic floor muscles can become damaged during delivery, creating weakness, which in turn can cause symptoms like incontinence. During delivery, tissue damage like tearing can also occur either in the levator ani muscles (the bowl of muscles that form the floor of the pelvis and play a starring role in urinary and bowel function, organ support, and posture), which are severely stretched during delivery, or in the perineum or anus, which can cause postpartum pain and/or dysfunction. If tissue is torn (skin can tear without necessarily tearing muscle), the scar it forms can create pain upon compression or stretching, such as with sex or exercise. The pudendal nerve will also be stretched, resulting in a tension injury to the nerve. In most cases, these nerve injuries recover; however, some lasting effects are common and can contribute to both fecal and urinary incontinence. Whew! Knowing what happens to the pelvic floor during childbirth makes it a bit easier to grasp how problems can arise postpartum. These problems include incontinence, both urinary and fecal; back, groin, hip, vulvovaginal, perineal, tailbone, or pelvic floor pain; pain during sex; diminished or absent orgasm; urinary frequency, urgency, or retention (retention is difficulty starting the urine stream); constipation and difficulty evacuating stool; and difficulty with exercise. In addition, a very common abdominal issue that arises postpartum is a diastasis recti, which is a separation of the rectus abdominis or "six-pack" abdominal muscles from their central tendon. This causes abdominal weakness and has been linked to incontinence and back pain in postpartum women. (See below for more details about diastasis recti.) Plus, as was already touched on, vaginal tearing or an episiotomy performed during a vaginal delivery can also cause future pelvic floor muscle problems. (A third- or fourth-degree vaginal tear has gone deep enough into the tissue to tear pelvic floor muscles.)

Pelvic floor PT can easily treat many of the issues listed above. Just as a hamstring tear or rotator cuff tear needs PT, the pelvic floor muscles need proper rehab after pregnancy/delivery. And pelvic floor PT can help even if years have gone by since a woman has given birth. Ideally, however, if a problem has persisted for three months postpartum, it's time to get help. But sadly, the majority of new moms in the United States have no idea that PT can help them. Indeed, postpartum recovery/rehab has not completely caught on in the United States. Other countries, like France, Denmark, Australia, and the United Kingdom are much more attuned to this health issue. Consider France. In France, it's the standard of care for every new mom to receive PT after she delivers a baby. Specifically, after giving birth, women are prescribed 10 to 20 sessions of *la rééducation périnéale*. Translation: "PT designed to strengthen and rehabilitate the muscles of the pelvic floor." Toward that end, physical therapists, or as they're referred to in France, *kinésithérapeutes*, use both manual, internal techniques and biofeedback to strengthen and rehabilitate a new mom's pelvic floor. In addition to these initial appointments focused on the pelvic floor, 10 additional visits are prescribed that are primarily aimed at treating the abdominal wall for diastasis recti issues. The main goal of the program, which was instituted in 1985 and is paid for by French Social Security, is to prevent postpartum incontinence and pelvic organ prolapse and to restore sexual function. And indeed, the absence of postpartum pelvic floor rehab has been linked to long-term issues, such as incontinence and organ prolapse. Here in the United States, a pelvic floor evaluation and PT postpartum is not part of our labor and delivery culture. Typically, as was the case with Angela, once a new mom has been cleared to begin having sex again after her six-week follow-up appointment, she's simply advised to do Kegels. (Frustratingly, studies show that 40% of women who are told to do Kegels by their health care providers aren't doing them correctly, so it would seem that verbal instruction isn't enough. Women need someone to show them, not just tell them, how to do a Kegel.)[3] However, inroads are being carved out in the United States as more doctors are starting to prescribe postpartum PT, more women are starting to request it, and more PTs are starting to offer it.

POSTPARTUM PELVIC FLOOR REHAB

We believe it's beneficial for all new moms to have their pelvic floor evaluated after they've been cleared to resume sex and exercise. This kind of early intervention can help address any concerns and ultimately enable new moms to return to functional and active lives, while possibly preventing future pelvic floor dysfunction. At our clinics we treat not only incontinence but also the myriad of other postpartum problems that can crop up. So when we see a postpartum patient, whether it's for incontinence or another postpartum concern, we work to uncover any and all postpartum issues she may be having. Toward that end, the initial evaluation for the postpartum patient includes:

- Musculoskeletal examination: This includes a manual evaluation of the pelvic floor muscles, where we can identify problematic muscles and scar tissue and develop a treatment plan based on our findings.
- Diastasis recti examination: See below for a detailed look at how a diastasis recti is corrected with pelvic floor PT.
- Scar mobilization for C-section, episiotomy, and other vaginal scars: Scar tissue can cause persistent pain and lead to discomfort and pain with intercourse. (See below for an in-depth look at C-section scar problems and solutions.)
- Manual PT for concerns of pain with vaginal intercourse or penetration: operative or vaginal delivery can result in tissue hypersensitivity around the episiotomy scar and/or any scar tissue from perineal trauma or tearing as well as create trigger points or tightness in traumatized muscle in and around the pelvic floor. Therefore, the PT will work to normalize pelvic floor muscle tone, eliminate trigger points, and decrease tissue hypersensitivity with manual techniques that can successfully resolve pain with vaginal intercourse or penetration.
- Pelvic floor muscle motor control exercises and training to treat urinary and/or fecal incontinence: Treating incontinence involves a host of exercises to strengthen the pelvic floor muscles as well as improve their motor control and endurance.

UNZIPPED: WHAT IS A DIASTASIS RECTI?

Most women seem to accept that pregnancy/childbirth changes their bodies. But what many don't realize is that some of these changes can be fixed. One of the "fixable" changes is a diastasis recti.

A diastasis recti is a separation of the rectus abdominis muscles, what many refer to as the "six-pack" muscles. This separation occurs along the band of connective tissue that runs down the middle of the rectus abdominis muscles. (This band of tissue is called the linea alba, but for our purposes, from here on out, we're going to refer to it as the midline.) During pregnancy, separation occurs down the midline because of the force of the uterus pushing against the wall of the abdomen coupled with the influx of pregnancy hormones that soften connective tissue.

A diastasis recti can occur anytime in the last half of pregnancy but most commonly occurs after pregnancy when the abdominal wall is lax and the thinner midline tissue no longer provides adequate support for the torso and internal organs. A small amount of widening of the midline happens in all pregnancies and is normal. Although some women's midlines spontaneously close after labor, for many, the tissue remains too wide. A midline separation of more than 2 to 2.5 finger widths, or 2 centimeters, is considered a problem. Predisposing factors for a diastasis recti include obesity, multiple births, and abdominal wall laxity from abdominal surgery.

What's the Problem with a Diastasis Recti?

A diastasis recti can lead to pelvic instability due to abdominal wall weakness. This instability can create a number of problems, including:

- Abdominal discomfort with certain movements, such as rolling over in bed, getting in/out of bed, and lifting heavy objects
- Umbilical hernia
- Pelvic girdle pain
- Sacroiliac joint pain
- Low back pain
- Pelvic floor dysfunction, such as urinary and fecal incontinence and pelvic organ prolapse

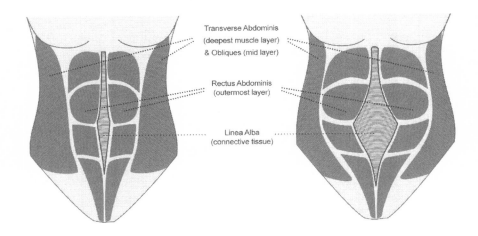

Figure 7.2.   Comparison of a normal abdomen verses an abdomen with a diastasis recti abdominus. *Source: MuTu System*

- Many new moms with a diastasis recti when they return to exercise might feel that they can't adequately perform certain exercises.
- In addition, a diastasis recti can change the appearance of the abdomen. The skin may droop, and some patients may even develop a hernia through the midline. Some postpartum patients with a diastasis recti complain of continuing to look pregnant.

Oftentimes patients want to know if they can do anything during pregnancy to prevent a diastasis recti. Our advice to them is to keep their abdominal muscles strong during pregnancy with appropriate exercises; maintain proper posture with sitting, standing, and activities such as pushing the grocery cart; avoid sit-up and double leg lift exercises; and avoid bearing down when doing activities such as lifting heavy objects and eliminating bowels. Aside from this, we teach patients proper techniques for getting up from a lying-down position as well as other general healthy body mechanics.

How Common Is a DR?

The reality is that about 53% of women have a diastasis recti immediately after delivery. This is because the tissues at the front of the abdomen are designed to allow the expansion of the belly in order to accommodate a growing baby. However, 36% of women will have a diastasis that remains abnormally wide at five to seven weeks postpartum.[4]

How Does One Check for Diastasis Recti?

The sooner a diastasis recti is caught, the easier it is to rehab. Here's how to check for a diastasis:

- Lie on your back with your knees bent and your feet on the floor.
- Place the fingertips of one hand at your belly button, and while your abdomen is relaxed, gently press your fingertips into your abdomen.
- Lift the top of your shoulders off the floor into a "crunch" position.
- Feel for the right and left sides of your rectus abdominis and take note of the number of fingers that fit into the gap.
- You will want to test this again approximately 1 to 2 inches above and below your belly button to determine the length of the gap.

If you find you have a diastasis, you will need to be cautious of the following activities, as they can create further separation of the abdominal muscles:

- abdominal sit-ups
- crunches
- oblique curls
- double leg lifts
- upper body twisting exercises
- exercises that include backbends over an exercise ball
- yoga postures that stretch the abs, such as "cow" pose and "updog" pose
- Pilates exercises that require the head to be lifted off the floor
- lifting and carrying heavy objects
- intense coughing without abdominal support

Basically, you will need to be cautious of any exercise that causes your abdominal wall to bulge out upon exertion. Once the diastasis is closed, you can gradually add these activities back in.

Diastasis Recti Correction

In general, correcting a diastasis includes core stabilization exercises, postural training, education on proper mobility techniques, and proper lifting techniques, as well as a fitting for an abdominal brace if needed (we will discuss this later on). In some cases, a self-guided program may be enough to correct a diastasis. But we recommend that postpartum women see a qualified pelvic floor PT if they believe they have a diastasis, because often other postpartum pelvic floor issues are at play. Here's a complete rundown of what we do to repair a patient's diastasis. During the first visit, we assess the length and width of the separation, the strength of the patient's abdominal muscles, the motor control of the pelvic floor, and the patient's posture. In addition, we assess hip, back, and sacral stability. Uncovering a patient's overall impairments is important in correcting a diastasis because only then can we put together a proper treatment plan. Since every patient is different, treatment plans are specifically tailored for each patient.

So how do we get down to actually closing the diastasis? Thankfully, closing a diastasis is not rocket science, and there are actually a few different methods for doing so. Here's our approach: the patient takes a towel or bedsheet, wraps it around her waist, and crosses it at the largest gap in the separation. For most people the largest gap is at the belly button. The patient must hold the sheet nice and tight, making sure the sheet is in between the ribs and hip bones, as they can hinder the sheet from being as tight as it needs to be. In that position, the patient does mini sit-ups. Patients need to do 30 to 60 daily repetitions of these sit-ups for a diastasis to close. Doing sit-ups without a towel or sheet could cause the gap to widen. But we'd like to stress that there are other approaches to closing a diastasis. Our advice to all new moms who believe they may have this issue is to seek out a health care professional for guidance. In addition to instructing patients on this exercise, we work to educate patients on what activities/exercises to do and not to do. For example, we'll tackle postural education, meaning we will show them how to sit and stand correctly; we teach them how to best carry heavy items (although this should be avoided if at all possible); how to lift objects correctly, including the baby; and how to correctly get into and out of bed, among other things.

As far as how long it takes for a diastasis to close, it all depends on the size of the gap, the amount of abdominal muscle strength, and other issues, such as obesity. The wider the gap, the longer rehabbing it will take. That said, although every patient is different, changes should start to occur within six weeks of rehab. But some patients do require surgery to correct a diastasis if it's not closing. If a patient doesn't see a sufficient closure in a 12-month time frame with consistent rehab efforts, then a surgical repair may be necessary. A general surgeon or a plastic surgeon can perform the surgery.

To Brace or Not to Brace

According to the social media/blogging world, *every* postpartum woman needs to wear a brace. This is simply incorrect messaging. So when is it appropriate to wear a brace? If a new mom can't reduce her diastasis through rehab and/or it's causing her significant daily limitations and pain, a brace may be useful. If a brace does provide comfort, it's a sign that the diastasis is a functional problem and should be addressed. In most cases it's okay to wear the brace for support while determining an effective course of treatment.

C-SECTION SCARS: PROBLEMS AND SOLUTIONS

A major issue that we treat for new moms involves C-section scarring. As of 2013, 32.7% of births ended in C-section.[5] "C-section" is short for cesarean section and is the delivery of a baby through an incision in the mother's abdomen and uterus. These days the most common incision used for a C-section is the "horizontal" or "bikini" incision. The incision is cut through the lower abdomen at the top of the pubic hair just over the hairline. Scarring from the incision builds up underneath the incision as well as in the uterus.

Now let's take a look at some potential problems caused by a C-section scar. A common complaint after a C-section is the sensitivity of the scar itself. For instance, it may hurt to lean over to pick up the baby or may cause pain with lifting or other positional changes. Standing up straight may be painful, as well as reaching over the head. In addition, the scar may cause a slight postural change, a sort of "pulling forward" that along with a decrease in the support of the back from the abdominal muscles could result in back pain. What's more, the round ligament that attaches from the sides of the uterus to the labia can be caught in scar tissue after a C-section because the incision is also right over the area where the round ligament crosses the pelvic brim. If this happens, a woman can experience labial pain, especially with transitional movements like going from a seated position to a standing position. Issues with lower digestion, such as irritable bowel syndrome or constipation, are also a possible consequence. This occurs because the scar tissue pulls within the abdominal cavity, affecting the organs. The good news is that the problems caused by a C-section scar can be treated with PT. *So how does a PT treat a C-section scar?* Most problems caused by C-section scarring can be improved or corrected altogether by making the scar more flexible by manipulating (moving and massaging) the scar tissue. The more scar tissue is moved and massaged, the softer and more similar to the tissue around it it becomes. This reduces tightness and breaks up adhesions (an adhesion occurs when scar tissue attaches to a nearby structure). Also, if a scar is pulled in all directions, the body will lay down the fibers of the scar tissue with more organization and in a similar alignment to the tissues around it. The scar blends in better and behaves more like normal tissue. So on the treatment table the PT will massage and manipulate your C-section scar and the area around it. Scars (internal and external) can be pushed, pulled, pinched, rolled, and rubbed. (Warning: manipulating a scar can be painful. That's because tissue that has restricted blood flow is super-sensitive to touch.) But this is a pain that comes with gain. Ultimately, scar mobilization promotes collagen remodeling, which increases pliability of the tissues and reduces uncomfortable sensations, such as itching or sensitivity. It's best to start C-section scar mobilization early in the healing process, usually six to eight weeks after the procedure. The reason early intervention is ideal is that the tissue will respond quickest during this period. However, the body remodels scar tissue constantly, so your tissues are being replaced with new tissue all the time, just at a much slower rate when scar tissue is older. A PT can also instruct a new mom how to perform the mobilization at home if appropriate.

"COMMON" BUT NOT NORMAL: INCONTINENCE AND PROLAPSE

Two of the most common postpartum problems new moms face either soon after giving birth or years later are incontinence and prolapse. First, let's take a look at incontinence. Postpartum women with urinary incontinence can leak urine when they sneeze, cough, laugh, or run. Some feel a frequent or sudden urge to urinate, even when their bladder isn't full. Others are unable to start the flow of urine at will or empty their bladder completely when urinating. Postpartum fecal incontinence is also possible. And many postpartum women have difficulty controlling gas or bowel movements. The main reason postpartum urinary incontinence occurs is damage to the muscles involved in continence. For example, muscle tearing during delivery or weakened, overstretched muscles can lead to incontinence. Also laughing, sneezing, coughing, jumping, running, or engaging in any activity that increases abdominal pressure places more pressure on the muscles that control continence, making them work harder. If they are weakened, they just can't do their job under increased pressure. Frustratingly, many women with incontinence postpartum do not seek help for their symptoms. That's because women often view urinary incontinence as either an unavoidable consequence of childbirth or a normal part of the aging process. Society validates these misconceptions in a number of ways; for instance, depicting new moms in all manner of media making light of how they "leak" every time they laugh or sneeze or by normalizing the condition with advertisements for "incontinence products." Plus, when a woman initially talks to her doctor about any problems she might be having with incontinence, she is simply told to "do Kegels." And as mentioned above, many women who do attempt to take this advice do the exercises incorrectly due to a lack of guidance. (Another issue with universally telling women with incontinence to "do Kegels" is that if the woman also has a tight pelvic floor, doing Kegels can cause pelvic pain. Plus, pelvic muscle weakness is not the only issue that causes incontinence, so muscle-strengthening exercises may be completely inappropriate.) In the case of postpartum women, muscle dysfunction or nerve injury causes incontinence; therefore, a PT would create an individualized program to correct whatever impairments are at play by increasing strength, coordination, and endurance of the pelvic floor and girdle

muscles. In rare instances muscle tightness is contributing to incontinence, and a PT would normalize the tone of the muscles, then check
motor control and teach strengthening if necessary.

Pelvic organ prolapse goes hand in hand with incontinence as a
major postpartum-related pelvic floor issue caused by a weakening of
the pelvic floor. Remember, one of the jobs of the pelvic floor is to
support the organs of the pelvis. But for a variety of reasons, and pregnancy is a major reason, the muscle and connective tissue that offer that
support can weaken. When they do, the organs can prolapse, descend-
ing into the vagina and causing a myriad of symptoms. This can happen
immediately after childbirth or slowly over time and may not be appar-
ent until a woman is older. (In women the pelvic organs include the
cervix, uterus, bladder, urethra, intestines, and rectum.) There are five
common types of prolapse into the vagina:

- Cystocele: the bladder descends into the vagina.
- Urethrocele: the urethra descends into the vagina.
- Rectocele: the rectum descends into the vagina.
- Enterocele: the small intestines descend into the vagina.
- Uterine prolapse: the uterus descends into the vagina.

While some prolapses can be asymptomatic, common complaints of
women with prolapse are inability to wear a tampon; urinary and/or
fecal incontinence; and pain with intercourse. As the pelvic organ prolapse gets worse, some women complain of:

- Pressure or a heavy sensation in the vagina that worsens by the
  end of the day or during bowel movements
- The feeling that they are "sitting on a ball"
- Needing to push stool out of the rectum by placing their fingers
  into or around the vagina during a bowel movement
- Difficulty starting to urinate or a weak or spraying stream of urine
- Urinary frequency or the sensation that they are unable to empty
  their bladder well
- Low back discomfort
- The need to lift up the bulging vagina or uterus to start urination
- Urinary leakage with intercourse

Like incontinence, prolapse is a common condition. Indeed, it's estimated that nearly 50% of all women between the ages of 50 and 79 have some form of prolapse.[6] In addition to childbirth, obesity and menopause are other factors that can contribute to developing a prolapse. *What are the treatment options for prolapse?* Lifestyle modifications and exercises for the pelvic floor muscles are typically the first line of treatment for the condition, both of which can be very effective. Lifestyle modifications include not straining with bowel movements and not lifting heavy items, and learning to avoid increasing abdominal pressure during daily activities. In some cases, wearing a pessary, which is a removable device that is placed into the vagina to help support the organ/organs from falling/bulging, is another nonsurgical way to manage a prolapse. Surgery is typically done only after a patient has tried conservative management first. In addition, a pelvic floor PT can help patients with prolapse by assessing the strength of the pelvic floor muscles and abdomen and also educating patients about specific strengthening routines that can help support the pelvic organs. Also, a PT can ensure that patients are not performing any lifting or other activities that will make a prolapse worse. Lastly, the PT can discuss whether a patient should see a physician for a surgical consult. *Can prolapse be prevented?* The answer to this is sometimes, but not always. That said, to attempt prevention, patients can avoid chronic straining, whether with exercise or when having a bowel movement; manage their weight; and maintain strength and stability in their pelvic floor and pelvic girdle muscles. Even if surgery is eventually needed to correct a prolapse, going into the surgery with a more normally functioning pelvic floor is only going to help matters. Look at it as the same as going into an ACL repair in the knee with strong surrounding muscles in the legs and hips versus weak muscles. However, when it comes to pelvic floor strengthening, we're hesitant to straight out advocate strengthening exercises, aka Kegels, because we are not in the business of recommending Kegels across the board for all the reasons we've already discussed. That said, if there is a true weakness (without muscle tightness or trigger points), then Kegels can help.

EXERCISE AFTER PREGNANCY

Most women are cleared for exercise at their six-week postpartum ob-gyn appointment. But as you've likely realized at this point in the chapter, postpartum recovery is complicated, and clearing every new mom for exercise six weeks after delivery perhaps isn't the best rule of thumb. That's because for a variety of reasons, not *all* new moms are ready to return to *all* exercise post-baby. For example, if there were any complications during delivery, or if a new mom isn't fully healed, which can mean many things, she may not be able to start exercising. Also, if a new mom still has a lot of hypermobility due to hormone changes and is feeling pain in her pelvis, pubic bones, or sacroiliac joint, she is probably not ready to jump back into exercise full force. Another example is a woman with a diastasis. As we've already explained, anyone with this issue should steer clear of core-heavy exercise, like Pilates, for instance. Factors that come into play when deciding whether a woman is ready to return to exercise after having a baby include:

- Her prior level of exercise. For instance, if the woman wasn't a runner prior to pregnancy, it's not a good idea to start running right after giving birth.
- What happened during delivery? For instance, did she have a vaginal delivery or a C-section? If she has an episiotomy scar or a C-section scar, she might have to wait longer than six weeks for the scar to heal.
- Are her joints still too mobile from all that relaxin that was released during pregnancy? Joints that are too mobile (a term we in the PT world refer to as hypermobile) can set someone up for injury.
- Is she breastfeeding? The hormones associated with breast milk cause ligaments to become lax (hypermobility).

In a perfect world, every postpartum woman would seek an evaluation from a PT to determine if/when and to what degree she is ready to return to exercise. But unfortunately we don't live in that world. So at the very least, it's our advice that if a new mom is having any pain, such as low back or pelvic girdle pain, or had any prepartum pain, musculoskeletal impairments are likely making postpartum exercise challenging, and a PT evaluation may be warranted. Frustratingly, we live in a society that puts an insane amount of pressure on new moms to get their pre-baby bodies back, fast! Not only are magazines filled with Photoshopped images of postpartum celebs with headlines shouting how so-and-so LOST ALL THAT BABY WEIGHT! but the message is even doled out from our family and friends. We ourselves may even be guilty of it. How many times has the first thing you've said to a family member or friend who's just given birth been, "Wow, you look great!" If you think about it, it's a strange thing to say to a woman who's been through the baby-birthing mill. Unfortunately, so many new moms succumb to this societal pressure and push themselves too hard upon their return to exercise post-baby. We've seen this time and again with our patients. Our advice to all new moms when returning to exercise postpartum is to really listen to your body. If you feel like you're pushing yourself too hard to perform an exercise post-baby, then nine times out of ten, you are. This is an instance where "pushing through the pain" is the wrong thing to do. And as we've already mentioned, urine leakage during exercise postpartum is a sign that there is a pelvic floor impairment that needs to be checked out by a PT. In addition, many postpartum women who return to exercise complain of having a hard time getting back into the swing of things; they might say "they don't feel it" or "they can't do it right" when they're doing certain exercises. This might be a red flag that musculoskeletal impairments, such as a diastasis recti, need to be corrected.

PREGNANCY CONCERNS FOR WOMEN WITH A HISTORY OF PELVIC PAIN

So many women who develop pelvic pain do so in the midst of their childbearing years, so they're faced with the prospect of getting pregnant and giving birth while recovering from or managing a pelvic pain syndrome. Many questions crop up for them when tackling this major life decision, one that is rife with unknowns in the best of circumstances. Two of the most common considerations for women recovering from or managing pelvic pain are: *Do I need to come off all my medication before trying to get pregnant?* and *How will any hormonal fluctuations that come along with pregnancy or any necessary fertility treat-*

ments affect my pelvic pain? We put these questions to one of our colleagues in treating pelvic pain, Sarah D. Fox, M.D., an ob-gyn who serves as an assistant professor of obstetrics and gynecology at the Warren Alpert Medical School of Brown University. Here's what Dr. Fox had to say about trying to get pregnant while managing pelvic pain with medication:

> Typically, medications are not studied in pregnant women—fewer than 10% of FDA-approved medications have been studied in human pregnancy—so there is much uncertainty about medication safety in pregnancy. That said, a few medications are well studied and safe (category A) and a few medications are not well studied in humans, but there is no evidence of harm in animal studies (category B) and these medications may be taken in pregnancy. However, the greatest number of medications fall into "category C," where there is evidence of risk to the fetus in animal studies, but there is no data in humans. But in some cases, the benefits of treatment may outweigh the risk to the fetus. For example, many of the antidepressants are category C drugs, so there may be some risk involved; however, we know that women who experience untreated depression in pregnancy can have adverse outcomes related to their depression. In some cases, women may be able to manage depression with counseling and behavioral changes. But in others with more severe symptoms, it may be better to continue the medication. Category D medications show that they are associated with increased fetal risks, but there may still be a compelling reason to use such medications. For example, benzodiazepines, such as Valium, which are sometimes used vaginally to treat pelvic pain, would fall into this category. Lastly, "category X" indicates that there is significant fetal risk, and these medications should not be used in pregnancy. It is very important to call and ask your obstetrician about your medications as soon as you realize you are pregnant. It is also important to remember that 50% of pregnancies in the United States are unplanned, and by the time the pregnancy is recognized, there will already be fetal exposure. It seems that many women with pelvic pain feel that their pain will prevent them from getting pregnant. Although this may be the case, it's important to realize that if you are not using contraception, you may become pregnant. If you are taking medications that fall into categories C, D, or X, it's best to make sure you are using contraception and you speak with your pain management physician and your ob-gyn before trying to become pregnant. Here is a great source of informa-

tion on medications and pregnancy from the Centers for Disease Control: http://www.cdc.gov/pregnancy/meds/index.html.[7]

When asked about how the hormonal changes that occur during pregnancy or any necessary fertility treatments, Dr. Fox explained:

> Hormonal changes that occur with pregnancy can certainly impact pelvic pain. For example, later in pregnancy there are elevations in the hormones estrogen and progesterone. For its part, the progesterone can actually be helpful in downregulating endometriosis, which may help make some women feel more comfortable during pregnancy. However, it also can be involved in causing laxity of the ligaments and joints. This is part of the mechanism by which women may experience pain in their pelvic girdle, SI joints, and pubic symphysis. In addition, progesterone levels (as well as the multivitamins and iron that many women take) can cause constipation that can worsen pelvic pain symptoms. And the mass effect of the pregnant uterus can cause worsening pain for many women, especially for those with bladder pain. Bladder pain may also worsen related to both the trauma of a vaginal delivery as well as after a C-section where the bladder is surgically manipulated. Also, with a 50% increase in blood volume during pregnancy, women experience more swelling, typically in the lower extremities. This swelling may worsen pelvic pain in some women. All that said, it is really challenging to predict how pregnancy will impact a woman's pelvic pain. Some women will feel better; others will feel worse during pregnancy and in the postpartum period. In any case, it is important not to get pregnant to improve pelvic pain, something that can backfire. For a pelvic pain patient who wants to have children, it is best to meet with your pain management physician before attempting pregnancy. This will allow you to determine all potential pain generators and examine which treatment options are available in pregnancy. It also allows you to set up resources for pregnancy, such as working with a pelvic floor PT to address the change in center of gravity, back pain, and pelvic girdle laxity.[8]

One question we as pelvic floor PTs get quite often from our patients who are considering getting pregnant is whether they should opt for a C-section or vaginal birth. Currently, no evidence exists to support whether one method of delivery is better than the other for a woman with pelvic pain. That said, if a woman has a pudendal nerve issue, is hypermobile, or suffered severe prolapse from a prior birth, a C-section may be recommended by a pelvic pain specialist. Our overall recommendation is for the patient to discuss this with her physician.

PHOEBE'S STORY

In the middle of the second trimester of my first pregnancy, I woke up one morning in terrible pain. It felt like I was being stabbed with a sharp knife in my bikini area. It hurt so badly that at times I could barely walk. Walking uphill or upstairs was extremely painful. I had to stop traveling for work. I actually got a handicap placard for my car because walking was so painful. Lying down was the only position that was comfortable. I had no idea what was happening, and I was terribly afraid I was going to have this pain for the rest of my pregnancy. I saw two doctors who diagnosed me as having "round ligament pain." They told me to take Tylenol and use a heating pad to help with the pain. It was my midwife who referred me to an orthopedic PT. The PT massaged my bikini area, and that helped to relieve the pain for short spurts of time; otherwise, I dealt with the pain for seven weeks, after which time it went away. But my relief was short-lived. In my third trimester, I began to notice that if I'd sit for long periods of time, my tailbone would begin to hurt. I remember being in the car during a long drive and being very uncomfortable. I found myself holding on to the bar on the roof of the car to ease the pressure on my tailbone area. At first I didn't really think much of the pain. I just figured it was a normal pregnancy issue. I went into labor about one month early. It was a pretty traumatic birth. I pushed for three hours. My son was eventually delivered via a vacuum-assisted vaginal delivery with an episiotomy. At about six weeks postpartum, I thought, "Oh my gosh! I'm still in a lot of pain down there!" It felt as if my pubic bone was bruised. It was pretty much in constant pain that would fluctuate in intensity. It especially worsened when I walked. And the tailbone pain I had noticed before my son was born was still there. Again, I turned to my midwife for advice. She referred me to PHRC for postpartum pelvic floor PT. In addition to focusing on my tailbone and pubic bone pain, Malinda, my PT at PHRC, also tackled the vaginal pain I was having as a result of my episiotomy and vacuum delivery. The scar tissue from the procedure was healing really hard and tough. It felt tight and sensitive down there. Sex was very painful. In addition, I was having some urinary incontinence. Malinda uncovered the impairments causing my pain, including a diastasis recti, a weak pelvic floor, hypersensitivity along my episiotomy scar, and connective tissue restrictions along my abdomen and pubic area. I gradually got better with twice-weekly PT sessions and with the help of the home treatment program Malinda prescribed, which included exercises to close my diastasis, self-massage with a tennis ball and foam roller for trigger points in my buttocks, episiotomy scar desensitization with dilators, and use of a support belt to help stabilize my pelvis. As we progressed in PT, she added exercises to strengthen my core and keep my hips in alignment. I went to PT for three months. It wasn't easy. The external work was pretty painful, although it did get less painful as time went on. That's where my history as an athlete really came in handy! I've been through hard training before, and I knew I could get through treatment. I wanted to have more children, so my goal was to fix my pelvic floor issues before my next pregnancy. After my experience, I've become a big advocate for pelvic floor PT for pregnancy. I tell my family members and friends who are pregnant that they should see a pelvic floor PT at least once to check things out with their pelvic floors. And to those who do have pain or other issues during pregnancy, I tell them they don't have to live with pain, and they shouldn't.

CONCLUSION

In this chapter we've covered the many issues associated with pregnancy and the pelvic floor, for women who are pregnant, new moms, and women with pelvic pain who are considering their reproductive options. In addition to pregnancy, another important function that is impacted by pelvic pain is sexual functioning. In the next chapter, we'll shine a light on exactly how pelvic pain can impact a person's sexual functioning.

8

PELVIC PAIN AND SEX: THE FACTS

As has already been discussed, the tissue, muscles, and nerves of the pelvic floor play a major role in sexual functioning. Therefore, it should come as no surprise that when impairments occur within the pelvic floor and surrounding tissue, sexual functioning is often impacted. To be sure, impaired sexual functioning is a common symptom of pelvic pain and can occur as a result of arousal, intercourse, orgasm, or post-orgasm. Symptoms of sexual pain and/or dysfunction can manifest in a number of different ways for someone with pelvic pain. For one thing, impaired tissue can be tender to the touch or can cause pain as a result of friction or compression. Pain can also occur as a result of orgasm or after orgasm due to the contraction of dysfunctional muscles or irritated nerves. Or sexual dysfunction can occur, such as erectile dysfunction in men due to too-tight muscles or restricted connective tissue or an in-ability to achieve orgasm in both sexes due to impaired muscles and/or nerves. Some of the more common symptoms of impaired sexual func-tioning with pelvic pain include vulvar/vaginal pain with vaginal pene-tration, pain in the genitals post-ejaculation, pain with orgasm, inability to orgasm, decreased lubrication in women, and erectile dysfunction. However, while many physiological mechanisms can cause sexual dys-function, emotional issues also go along with pelvic pain and can also impact sexual functioning. For example, many people with pelvic pain become so used to viewing the pelvic floor as the source of their pain that they struggle to connect that part of their body with sexuality and pleasure. In this chapter, we're going to cover all these issues and more.

We'll begin the chapter with a brief overview of male and female sexual pain and dysfunction. Then we'll take a look at the role sexual function has in the PT treatment room. Finally we'll end the chapter with a discussion of some of the emotional issues that surround the impact of pelvic pain on sexual functioning.

MALE SEXUAL PAIN/DYSFUNCTION

For Billy, his sexual dysfunction was a symptom of a larger pelvic floor issue. At 32 he had been an avid cyclist for nearly 15 years. When he decided to compete in a triathlon, he upped his riding by 20 miles a week. Unfortunately, more time on his bike resulted in pelvic pain. Specifically, he began having right-side buttock pain and perineum pain. In addition, he developed erectile dysfunction that didn't respond to medication. Ultimately Billy made his way to PHRC for therapy with Stephanie. Stephanie found trigger points in his superficial pelvic floor muscles that were causing his perineum pain and erectile dysfunction, connective tissue restrictions in his buttocks causing his buttock pain, and lastly, a tight obturator internus muscle. Most likely a combination of all these impairments contributed to his erectile dysfunction. After about six months of PT, Billy's symptoms cleared up, including his erectile dysfunction.

Billy's case is but one example of the many ways pelvic pain can impact a male patient's sexual functioning. Below is a list of some of the other more common symptoms of sexual pain/dysfunction that can occur with pelvic pain along with a brief description of the possible physiological mechanisms behind each. Note: this is not meant to be a definitive list.

- perineal pain during intercourse or masturbation with thrusting due to perineal compression when there are trigger points in the perineum
- perineum or genital pain after sexual activity due to pelvic floor or girdle muscle trigger points or nerve irritation
- pain with ejaculation due to bulbospongiosus or ischiocavernosus trigger points or nerve irritation

- pain with touch anywhere on the genitals with manual stimulation or with a partner due to pudendal, sacral, or central nervous system irritation
- hypersensitivity (meaning light touch feels very irritating) at the tip of the penis due to pudendal, sacral, or central nervous system irritation
- lower abdominal, suprapubic, or bladder pain before, during, or after orgasm due to referred pain from the pelvic floor muscles, urethral irritation, or abdominal muscle trigger point
- decreased force of ejaculate due to tight pelvic floor muscles

Erectile Dysfunction and Pelvic Pain

A variety of things, such as cardiovascular disease, diabetes, obesity, or emotional issues can cause erectile dysfunction (ED). However, for a small percentage of men with ED, the pelvic floor may be the culprit. It's worth exploring the possibility that the pelvic floor is causing a man's ED in two situations. One, if the man's ED began around the same time as other pelvic floor symptoms/dysfunction, as was the case with Billy. And two, if all other possibilities and first-line treatments for ED have been tried and ruled out. To understand how the pelvic floor can cause ED, it helps to understand the role it plays in erection and ejaculation: First, blood rushes to the penis upon arousal. Then the ischiocavernosus (a pelvic floor muscle located at the base of the penis) contracts to keep the blood in the penis and maintain the erection. During sexual activity, the bulbospongiosus muscle (one of the superficial muscles of the pelvic floor) contracts and relaxes to push the ejaculate out.

If any of the aforementioned muscles are impaired, the process can be impacted. In addition, those muscles are innervated by part of the pudendal nerve. Therefore, if that nerve is impaired, it could negatively affect the performance of those muscles, again impacting the process. And in general, any pelvic floor impairment that affects healthy blood flow through the arteries involved in erection and ejaculation, like restricted connective tissue along the bony pelvis, can play a role in ED. On top of all that, painful contraction of those muscles during sex may also affect a man's ability to maintain an erection for psychological reasons.

FEMALE SEXUAL PAIN/DYSFUNCTION

Jessica, a 30-year-old patient of Liz, is an example of a patient whose sole symptom was pain with sex. She had been dating the same guy for seven years. The couple had never had intercourse because it was simply too painful for Jessica, not to mention that her muscles were so tight, her boyfriend's penis physically could not penetrate her vagina. Jessica was even unable to tolerate a gynecological exam with a speculum. Her condition is called vaginismus and is caused by involuntary spasming of the pelvic floor muscles surrounding the vagina. When Liz examined Jessica, she found that she did indeed have extremely tight pelvic floor muscles. Her approach to treating Jessica involved two main strategies: internal work to loosen Jessica's tight muscles and the use of dilators to desensitize the tissue. As a result of the manual treatment with Liz and the at-home dilator use, Jessica was ultimately able to have pain-free intercourse. Vaginismus is just one of many ways pelvic floor neuromuscular impairments can cause sexual pain/dysfunction in women. Below is a list of some other examples. Again, this is not meant to be a definitive list.

- vestibular/vulvar pain during intercourse or after intercourse, which can be caused by a number of neuromuscular issues, including too tight pelvic floor muscles or referred pain from pelvic floor muscle trigger points. It should also be pointed out that underlying causes besides neuromuscular impairments can play a role in vestibular/vulvar pain during intercourse, such as fissures and hormone imbalance. Additionally, the skin of the vulva and vestibule itself can be a source of pain. (Note: when the pain comes from the vestibule, the problem is referred to as provoked vestibulodynia.)
- vaginal pain during intercourse due to either too-tight pelvic floor muscles, pelvic floor muscle trigger points, or irritated pelvic floor nerves
- clitoral pain due to dermatological or hormonal issues, referred pain from pelvic floor muscles, or nerve hypersensitivity
- painful orgasm due to trigger points in the superficial pelvic floor muscles or nerve irritation

- Urinary urgency, frequency, and/or burning due to friction on the urethra and surrounding tissues or referred pain from the pelvic floor, pelvic girdle, or abdominal muscles

Persistent Genital Arousal Disorder

As you have realized by now, a number of different neuromuscular issues can impact a woman's sexual functioning; some, like vestibulodynia and vaginismus, have well-known diagnoses attached to them. Another diagnosis we would like to highlight in our discussion of female sexual pain/dysfunction is persistent genital arousal disorder, or PGAD. The International Society for the Study of Women's Health (ISSWSH) defines PGAD as "a persistent or recurrent, unwanted or intrusive, bothersome or distressing, genital dysesthesia (abnormal sensation) that is not associated with sexual interest." In other words, women with PGAD either constantly or periodically feel like they are on the verge of an orgasm in nonsexual places and times. They are unable to turn this feeling on or off. Normal sexual response has been defined as a four-stage cycle: excitement, plateau, orgasm, and resolution. People suffering from PGAD are thought to exist in the stages between excitement and orgasm, with no resolution. Symptoms can be associated with overactive bladder and restless legs syndrome, and for some sufferers achieving orgasm only further aggravates symptoms. (While the condition is thought to be more common in women, both men and women can suffer with PGAD.) An important thing to understand about PGAD is that the symptoms are not pleasurable, but painful. Although symptom severity varies among sufferers, this condition can be devastating for people. Patients we've treated who have PGAD have described the feeling as "extremely embarrassing, distracting, and painful." "It is impossible to interact socially and professionally with feelings of arousal. Medical professionals and well-intended friends and family members think it's funny or say they are 'jealous.' They have no idea what I am going through," explained one patient we have treated. It's only in the last few years that research has shed light on this perplexing problem. The current thought is that the symptoms of PGAD can be caused by excessive sensory peripheral information from irritated muscles, nerves, and/or genital tissues and/or a central sexual reflex that is under decreased inhibition from the central nervous system. *What causes a per-*

son to develop symptoms of PGAD? Exactly what causes PGAD is currently unknown. In a recent study of 15 women, symptoms of genital pain, depression, and interstitial cystitis were found in more than one-half of the patients. In addition, previous antidepressant use, restless legs syndrome, and pudendal neuralgia were found in a number of cases. Pelvic congestion syndrome and Tarlov cysts (fluid-filled sacs that most often affect nerve roots at the lower end of the spine) have been previously identified as possible contributors to PGAD, but these were not a common finding in this particular study.[1]

Currently PGAD is diagnosed based on a patient's symptoms, and a limited number of physicians in the United States have experience with PGAD. These physicians can be found through ISSWSH. As far as treatment goes, numerous interdisciplinary treatment combinations are considered reasonable options for people with PGAD. These include PT, TENS treatment, hypnotherapy, pharmaceutical management, hormonal regulation, pudendal nerve blocks, sympathetic nerve blocks, Botox, and neuromodulation.

PT AND SEXUAL HEALTH

As PTs, when we treat patients for pelvic pain–related symptoms, we pay attention to their sexual function. To be sure, when we interview patients in their first evaluation appointment, we always ask them questions about their sexual functioning, such as:

- *Is sex painful? If so, where exactly?*
- *When is it painful? (For instance, at the beginning during penetration or afterward or only during certain positions or only with intercourse or masturbation?)*
- *If it's a woman, is the pain superficial or deep?*
- *Has your ability to orgasm changed?*
- *If it's a woman, do you feel like you're producing adequate lubrication?*
- *If it's a man, is there pain during or after ejaculation?*
- *If it's a man, has the quality of your erection changed? Is it weaker now versus before your pelvic floor symptoms started?*

The responses to these questions can guide us as PTs in a myriad of ways. For example, if a male patient complains of pain with sitting or perineum pain, and he also has sexual dysfunction, we'll ask him if it started at the same time his pain started. If his answer is yes, that tells us his sexual dysfunction could be musculoskeletal in nature, so during our evaluation we'll home in on the pelvic floor muscles responsible for erection and ejaculation. For a female patient, if we uncover vulvar pain with penetration, we'll examine her more superficial muscles. Conversely, if she only complains of pain deeper with thrusting during sex, we'll focus on the deeper pelvic floor muscles, such as her levator ani muscle group or her obturator internus muscles. Two other important issues for us to consider when treating patients with sexual pain/dysfunction are hormones, especially for female patients, and what medications the patient is taking. Indeed, many different medications can affect sexual function. For instance, certain blood pressure medications cause erectile dysfunction. As for hormones, as we've already discussed in earlier chapters, for women, hormonal imbalance of estrogen and/or progesterone and/or testosterone can make sex painful or can interfere with the production of lubrication.

Will Sex Make My Pain Worse?

We often get this question from our patients, whether sex is painful for them or not, and the answer is not always a simple yes or no. For instance, we had a male patient whose penile pain, which was caused by trigger points in the ischiocavernosus and bulbospongiosus muscles, did intensify after sex and/or masturbation. So understandably, he was concerned that sexual activity was making his pain worse, and he wanted to know if he should discontinue having sex altogether. As a general rule, we rarely tell our patients to discontinue sexual activity, because the benefits can outweigh any negatives. For instance, the intimacy achieved with sex with a partner; the release of stress masturbation can achieve; and the overall endorphin rush sex produces all have benefits that can help someone with persistent pain. So it really is a personal decision for a patient to make: whether the benefit he/she gets from sexual activity is worth potentially slowing healing. All that said, there are two particular situations where a patient should be cautious. One, if a woman is experiencing vulvar tearing or fissuring every time she has penetration, it is important to treat whatever underlying problem is causing this prior to resuming intercourse. Also, patients should be aware that having sex "through the pain" may cause them to identify sex with pain, and that could set them up for avoidance issues that may interfere with sexual activity even after their pain resolves.

Lastly, a word on masturbation. When pelvic floor muscles become too tight, it's not uncommon for diminished orgasm to occur. As a result, it can be more difficult or take longer to achieve orgasm during masturbation. Therefore, patients report that they have to masturbate "more often" or "harder" to have an orgasm. Over the years, we've had quite a few patients who have told us they "over-masturbated" because their pain began shortly afterward and they feel guilty and ashamed. We always reassure them that they did not cause their pain by masturbating. We tell them that their impairments were lurking just below the surface and they would have become symptomatic eventually, whether they masturbated or not.

THE EMOTIONAL SIDE

Above we presented an overview of the physiological side of the impact pelvic pain has on sexual functioning; this section is devoted to a discussion of the emotional side. To present this side of the story, we thought it best to pick the brains of three top experts in sex therapy: Heather Howard, Ph.D., a board-certified sexologist and founder of the Center for Sexual Health and Rehabilitation in San Francisco; Rose Hartzell, Ph.D., a certified sex educator and therapist at San Diego Sexual Medicine; and Erica Marchand, Ph.D., a licensed psychologist specializing in couples and sex therapy in Los Angeles. In our discussions with these three experts, two major themes came up time and again. For one thing, many who deal with pelvic pain feel "broken" or "damaged." Secondly, oftentimes these folks end up avoiding intimacy altogether because of their pain.

Feeling "Broken"

A common emotional issue that comes up with pelvic pain patients around sex is feeling "broken" or feeling like less of a man or a woman.

"It's a loss of identity because so often people equate their manhood or womanhood with sexual functioning," explains Dr. Howard.[2] And with the societal weight placed on this part of the human anatomy, is it any wonder people can feel this way?

Getting Past Feelings of Brokenness

So what are some strategies that can help folks get past those feelings of "being broken"? One strategy is to "normalize" what is going on with the person and to work on overcoming feelings of isolation, says Dr. Howard. "One way of doing that is to explain that these are normal feelings for people with pelvic pain conditions," she says. Another big part of normalizing the situation is educating patients about exactly what's going on with their bodies from a physiological standpoint. In addition, if someone is in a partnered relationship and they fear their relationship will fail because of their "inadequacies," Dr. Howard reminds them "that all partnerships are going to hit stumbling blocks." Again, this helps the patient understand that they're not "broken" or "damaged" and that what they're going through with their partner is one of many challenges that can come up in a relationship.[3] Dr. Marchand agrees, explaining that all too often, people she works with take on an extraordinary amount of guilt for not being able to "satisfy their partners" sexually because of their pelvic pain issues, even going so far as to describe themselves as "freaks." The reality is, it's a pretty safe bet that all human beings will experience challenges in their sexual functioning, whether due to emotional issues, daily life stressors, health-related issues, or the normal results of aging. This is not to diminish what folks dealing with pelvic pain go through; it's simply a way to put the experience in perspective and help them feel less isolated and alone.

But for some, their feelings of being broken or damaged can shut down their sexuality. It's easy to understand why, says Dr. Marchand. So often, people begin to view the part of their body that once was an area of pleasure as an area that causes them pain and needs medical intervention. "So it becomes something that you don't associate with pleasure anymore," she says. "I don't want my patients to permanently associate their pelvic region with pain and medical intervention. So I think it's important to reclaim your genitals as an area of pleasure."

Some patients, such as women with vaginismus who have yet to have pain-free intercourse, might be doing this for the first time, points out Dr. Marchand. Toward this end, Dr. Marchand counsels patients to engage in masturbation or solo stimulation as a way to reconnect with this part of their body. "I will often counsel people to set aside some time and get comfortable, whether it's in your bed or on your couch or even on the floor on some pillows in front of a full-length mirror. I tell them not to answer their phones and to lock their doors. I ask them to get a mirror so they can see what they're doing. Then I ask them to use their fingers (skin on skin is better for this exercise than a vibrator) to explore their genitals. I want them to see what feels good to the touch, and what feels bad, both externally and internally. Having this level of awareness will not only help them reclaim this area of their body for pleasure, it'll also help them feel more in control when they're being intimate with a partner. To be sure, they'll be able to direct their partner on what to avoid and what kind of touch is pleasurable for them."[4]

TURNING OFF: INTIMACY AVOIDANCE

With pelvic pain, avoidance of sex or any intimacy at all is another common emotional issue. "For many of my patients, there is a fear that any type of physical touch will lead to intimacy or sexual intercourse; therefore, they'll close off all physical touch with their partner," explains Dr. Hartzell. "Ultimately, the physical distance will lead to emotional distance, and this can be disastrous for a relationship." And it can work both ways, she adds. She tells of a patient with vulvar pain who had a high sex drive, and on the days when she felt good enough to have sex, her partner was not interested because he had developed low sexual desire as a result of their complicated intimacy issues. His worry was always, "What if we are intimate, but she has pain, and there is a failed encounter?" Dr. Hartzell explained.[5] While everyone places a different weight on sex, and no one is saying that putting sex on the back burner is a good or bad thing, there can be negative consequences to turning off all physical touch, especially when you're in a relationship, points out Dr. Marchand. "It's possible for resentment or frustration to build up, which can be detrimental to the relationship," she says.[6] However, it's important, adds Dr. Howard, for those who go through this type of avoidance issue to understand that it's a "normal mechanism to back away from touch, because we as humans learn efficiently. And one of the first things that we learn is that pain is to be avoided. So it's really a functional response to someone's condition, not a dysfunctional one. The good news is that just as that behavior can be learned, it can be unlearned when a person with pelvic pain desires closeness and sexual contact with a partner. It is possible to break the association between pleasurable contact and pain."[7]

TURNING INTIMACY BACK ON

So how can someone dealing with pelvic pain overcome intimacy avoidance issues? "Because every patient/couple is unique, there is no standard," explains Dr. Hartzell. "Having said that, I will say that I always want to instill in my patients that there is no such thing as failed sex. Sex is not a performance, it's about having a connection, it's about fun, and it's about being intimate with your partner. And you can do that a lot of different ways. Often when I begin working with a couple I will try to take whatever activity is the most painful—and more often than not it's penetration—off the table. The goal is to get them to a place where instead of associating sex with pain, they begin to once again associate it with pleasure. The next step is to get them to be intimate again even if they can't have penetration or engage in other activities that are too painful. You would be surprised at how many people, especially women, are hung up on the idea that to have sex you must have penetration. The bottom line is sex does not equal penetration. There are so many other activities on the menu! For example, using a vibrator on the clitoris, oral sex, and clitoral stimulation without touching the vulva or the vagina, to name a few. I would like to add that this is also true for gay and lesbian couples dealing with sexual pain issues. *Penetration does not equal sex.*

"In addition, I'll often give my patients assignments to help them reestablish intimacy. One of my favorite assignments is for them to go to the dollar store to purchase $10 worth of items. Then each time they are intimate, they'll use one of the items. You would be surprised how much fun you can have with whipped cream or a spatula! Plus, I'm a big advocate of vibrators, so I have them go to a sex shop together and pick out one that they like, and begin experimenting with it. Also I ask them to participate in what is called 'sensate focus.' Here's how it works: the couple will set up their bedroom for intimacy—for example, lighting candles, putting on soft music—and then they'll get undressed, and each will spend 15 minutes or so giving the other pleasure, not orgasm, but exploring their partner's body. The partner on the receiving end is to give feedback as to what he or she likes/doesn't like. The communication is the key to this exercise. Oftentimes when you're caught up in the heat of sex, you're not going to 'spoil the moment' by telling your partner what's working or what's not working. But this way you're given the opportunity to really communicate what you like or don't like. Also, since the end goal is not about achieving orgasm, the pressure is off."[8]

EXPLAINING YOUR PAIN TO A POTENTIAL PARTNER

We've talked about how to communicate issues surrounding pelvic pain and sexual functioning with partners, but what about the impact your pelvic pain has on your sexual functioning as a single man or woman? How can you communicate your situation to a *potential* partner? Dr. Howard has some solid advice on this front. "My advice isn't so much concerning the words that you should use when you talk to a potential partner, it's more about coming from a place of self-worth when talking to that person. If you come into the conversation from an empowered space, as someone who sees him or herself in a positive light, who is a competent, successful person navigating a difficult health condition, you're less likely to overwhelm the person. Furthermore, it's important to come from a place of 'this is a part of me' as opposed to 'this is all of me' or 'this defines me.' So the more you approach it as a teacher, rather than someone begging for forgiveness, the greater the chance that the person feels like, 'Okay, I can learn something from you. You are clearly managing and living your life through this. You're moving along and you're doing okay, I guess I can be with you.' But if you speak as if you're not functioning, that's a lot for someone to want to take on."[9]

SUGGESTED READING FROM OUR THREE SEXUAL PAIN EXPERTS

- *Full Catastrophe Living* by Jon Kabat-Zinn is about a mind-body program for living with pain.
- *When Things Fall Apart* by Pema Chodron is about dealing with negative emotions without getting overwhelmed by them.
- *When Sex Hurts* by Andrew Goldstein and colleagues is great for information about sexual pain.
- *Guide to Getting It On* by Paul Joannides, *The New Male Sexuality* by Bernie Zilbergeld, and *The Elusive Orgasm* by Vivienne Cass all offer great insight and strategies for sexual exploration, especially when your sexual functioning has changed.
- Free sexual pain guides for patients and partners from the Center for Sexual Health and Rehabilitation can be found at http://sexualrehab.com/Additional-Resources.html.

SEXUAL PAIN: MELISSA'S STORY

I first noticed something was wrong when I tried to have sex with my boyfriend, now husband, for the first time and we were unable to have intercourse because it was extremely painful. I originally thought it was because I hadn't had sex in about a year—you know, "if you don't use it you lose it." But we tried a couple more times, and things didn't improve. After about a month, I began to realize I had a problem. Every time I would have sex, my perineum would tear, causing fissures. It was kind of like an unwanted episiotomy, but not as severe. First I went to my gynecologist, who I really loved. And her diagnosis was that I was having sex wrong. All my love for her faded in about 30 seconds, and I decided to leave her practice. When I went to see a second doctor, I brought photos I had taken of the tears. This second doctor allowed me to talk for less than a minute, looked at one of the pictures, and said that I had lichen sclerosus. I had actually come across this diagnosis in my research, so I knew what the symptoms were; therefore, I was doubtful, since they didn't sound like what I was experiencing. But she was convinced and proposed doing a biopsy to prove it. I agreed. So she did a biopsy of the tissue. But when I went in for my follow-up, she said she hadn't gotten enough tissue to confirm the diagnosis, but she was still positive that's what I had. At this point I'm thinking, "She's a doctor, she knows, and it's better to have a diagnosis rather than not know what's wrong with me." So I started steroid treatment, but deep down in my heart I knew I didn't have lichen sclerosus. Sex continued to be painful, and I could only tolerate it about once every one or two months. About a year later, a move caused me to have to switch doctors. I should also mention that I was going to the gynecologist rather frequently at this point because I was suffering from regular yeast and urinary tract infections. This cycle had started when I came down with a UTI but mistook the symptoms for my normal pain issues. When I finally went to a doctor and was diagnosed with a UTI, the infection was extremely bad and set me up for a vicious cycle of further UTIs and yeast infections. The next doctor's proposed treatment for the pain I was having with sex was to surgically remove the offending tissue and see if healthy tissue would grow back in its place. I looked at her and I said, "Have you done this before?" And she said, "Only once, and it didn't work. But we can try it." I thanked her for her time, and in my mind I said, "You will never see me again." So now I'm on to Doctor Number Four. I saw this doctor for about two years, and while she didn't believe that I had lichens (a subsequent biopsy showed that I indeed did not), she didn't have an explanation for the tearing and my pain with sex. Even though she didn't have any answers for me, I liked that she didn't offer any crazy theories or treatment. Things got a little better with time. I'd still tear, and there'd still be pain, but it wasn't as intense. I felt like I was in a kind of holding pattern. During that time I also had begun to see a naturopath, which didn't impact the tearing and pain, but I do believe it helped with the yeast infections and UTIs. I got engaged but decided to put my marriage plans on hold. I just got to thinking, what's the point of getting married if I could barely consummate it? I was getting tired of the entire situation. And so was my fiancé. We were both frustrated by the lack of answers. So I began thinking about visiting an out-of-state specialist. Ultimately, I went to see Doctor Number Six, a vulvodynia specialist in-state, but in another city. Upon examining me, he said: "Wow! You're very tight!" Then he explained what he believed had been happening to me. He said I had extremely tight pelvic floor muscles, so tight that they were pulling the skin of my vulva taut—kind of like a rubber band—causing the skin to tear during sex. After hearing this I began to cry with relief. "OKAY!" I thought. "This is an explanation I haven't heard before!" The doctor prescribed PT. Prior to traveling to see the vulvodynia specialist, I had begun to have other symptoms. Specifically, my vulvar tissue had begun to get really red, irritated, and itchy. I had started seeing a dermatologist for these symptoms. She had diagnosed me as having "vulvar eczema" and had prescribed various creams. So at this point, my thinking was that between the treatments the vulvodynia specialist and dermatologist had prescribed, I was on the road to recovery. I was so relieved to finally have answers and a plan that seemed to make sense. About one year and two PTs (the first didn't help at all, and the second did help a bit) later, things began looking up. I started feeling better. Most importantly, the tearing had pretty much gone away. The pain with sex improved as a result. I had started seeing a therapist, so my mental health had also started to improve. So I was feeling like things were on the upswing. Although I still had some pain with sex and zero sex drive, I could go through the motions and tolerate sex more often than once every few months. I didn't flinch every time my husband touched me, and I could actually achieve orgasm. So even though sex wasn't great, it was okay. I was dealing with it. My husband was dealing with it. We were managing. Then it occurred to me after watching a motivational speaker on television one night that I had gotten complacent with my recovery. Suddenly I began to want more than just "okay" out of my sex life. I wanted "great"! That's when I started seeing Stephanie for regular PT. What Stephanie found were extremely tight pelvic girdle muscles and connective tissue restriction, which were not previously examined/treated by the other two PTs I saw. My pelvic floor muscles were not as impaired as these other two areas, because those had received attention from the other PTs. She believed that my lack of sex drive was possibly due to a lack of blood flow to my genitals due to my muscles being so tight as well as long-term birth control use. I didn't cry this time, but hearing this from Stephanie was another feeling of epiphany. The funny thing is, throughout my life I have had plenty of people tell me my body is tight, from my husband to masseuses to PTs. To address this overall tendency for my muscles to become tight, Stephanie helped me figure out a plan to do regular yoga. Now I have sex without pain and I can orgasm on a regular basis. For me the final roadblock was the lack of arousal. Ultimately, I chose to replace the birth control pill with an IUD. About a month later, my arousal returned.

CONCLUSION

In this chapter we've provided an overview of how pelvic pain can impact healthy sexual functioning, from both a physiological perspective and an emotional one. It's a part of the pelvic pain story that highlights the need for patients to be active members of their treatment teams, a theme that we go into in much further detail in the next section of the book, beginning with the next chapter, where we tackle at-home self-treatment as part of an overall treatment plan.

III

In the Driver's Seat: Taking Control of Your Healing

9

AT-HOME SELF-TREATMENT: TAKING MATTERS INTO YOUR OWN HANDS

Many people dealing with pelvic pain (and likely many that are reading this book) have tried the different do-it-yourself "protocols" out there for treating their pain without success or even to the detriment of their symptoms. But when it comes to self-treatment, like most things having to do with pelvic pain recovery, there is no "one-size-fits-all" approach. To be sure, what might help one could harm another, even if symptoms are identical. Case in point: two women, we'll call them Leah and Sue, both suffer from daily vulvar burning. It's determined by their PT evaluations that both have tight hamstrings and tight hip external rotators (the small muscles of the hip that rotate the femur in the hip joint). Stretching these muscles has the potential to be helpful, but it would be a mistake to prescribe those stretches to both Leah and Sue. Here's why: it turns out Leah also has trigger points in her hamstring muscles as well as irritation of her posterior femoral cutaneous nerve (a nerve distributed to the skin of the perineum and the back surface of the thigh and leg) as primary drivers of her symptoms. So hamstring stretches could irritate her trigger points and further irritate her angry nerve. As for Sue, she *can* stretch her tight hamstrings no problem, but stretching her hip external rotators could activate the trigger points she has in her obturator internus muscles. Case in point: therapeutic exercise intended to treat one impairment, in these cases a muscle, can irritate other muscles, nerves, and joints. However, while there is no one-size-fits-all approach to at-home self-treatment, what can be beneficial to a patient's recovery is an *individualized* home program that's developed and supervised by a PT. Think about it: typically, patients will see their PTs for one-hour appointments each week. That's four hours a month—four hours out of approximately 720 hours a month! The right home program, while it won't heal patients' pelvic pain, has the potential to make them feel better while hastening recovery. Lastly, an added benefit to establishing an individualized home program is that it gives patients lifelong tools to manage flare-ups.

Because home programs are important in pelvic pain recovery, we've decided to devote this chapter to the topic with the resounding caveat that *patients use the information in this chapter to further the dialogue with their PT about their home programs as opposed to trying any of the suggestions on their own.* We'll begin the chapter by taking a general look at how a home program can help with recovery. Then we'll discuss the importance of timing in putting a program into action. Next we'll give some general advice for home treatment. Lastly, we'll end the chapter by discussing the one activity, so-called "pelvic floor drops," that does have a place in every home treatment program.

HOW HOME TREATMENT CAN HELP

"Home treatment" means different things to different patients. For instance, some of our patients manually treat themselves either internally (using a dilator, handheld wand, or their finger), externally, or both. In addition, patients do an individualized combination of stretches and strengthening exercises at home. Others bring their partner to a PT session so he/she can learn how to administer appropriate techniques, either internally, externally, or both, between PT sessions. What all home treatment programs have in common is that they're designed to help a patient reach his/her treatment goals. For instance, if a PT identifies a muscle as tight or weak, the PT can recommend specific exercises to help strengthen or lengthen the muscle. For example, many of our male patients have tight hamstring muscles (in fact, male hamstrings are 15% tighter than those of females), and this can affect how they sit, which can in turn cause or exacerbate their pelvic pain symptoms. Once the PT determines that the hamstring muscles are free of trigger points, hamstring stretches may be appropriate for such a patient. In addition, patients can treat tight external muscles as well as external trigger points, like trigger points in the gluteal muscles or inner thighs, with different tools. For example, we often teach our patients how to use a foam roller to help loosen tight muscles early in their treatment. (More on home treatment tools below.)

TIMING MATTERS

When putting together a home treatment program for a patient, timing plays a key role. What we mean by this is that certain home treatment techniques need to be phased in at certain points in a patient's recovery, not before. For this phasing-in process, we'd like to share a few general rules of thumb:

1. Begin to stretch too-tight muscles only when any trigger points in those muscles are gone and any nerves involved in symptoms and particular exercise have regained normal mobility. For instance, if hamstrings are tight and need to be stretched but have active trigger points and/or the posterior femoral cutaneous nerve (a nerve that runs through the hamstrings) is irritated, stretching this muscle could both aggravate the trigger points and inflame the posterior femoral cutaneous nerve, causing further nerve irritation and more symptoms. For patients who have too-tight muscles with trigger points and/or nerve irritation that's preventing them from doing stretches, one option to loosen those too-tight muscles is foam rolling.

2. Begin to strengthen any pelvic floor muscles once trigger points are gone, muscles are no longer too tight, and they are actually weak. As we've explained in previous chapters, too-tight muscles and/or muscles with trigger points can also have a problem with weakness. These muscles will need to be strengthened, but not until after trigger points have been eradicated and too-tight muscles have been returned to a healthy tone. For example, if a woman presents postpartum with urinary incontinence, sacroiliac joint pain, and pain with intercourse, and her PT finds both internal and external trigger points (causing the pain with intercourse) as well as overall pelvic floor weakness (contributing to the incon-

tinence), the PT is going to tackle the trigger points first, then incorporate exercises aimed at improving the strength and motor control of her pelvic floor muscles.

3. Doing internal work to treat trigger points or too-tight muscles could be counterproductive if certain other impairments exist, such as fissures, tissue that is lacking in estrogen, or irritated vestibular tissue. While the internal work might help with the trigger points or too-tight muscles, the benefit is often undone if it further irritates the aforementioned impairments.

HOME TREATMENT TIPS

In addition to advice on timing, a few other general tips can help make a home treatment program successful.

Tools can help.

A handful of different tools can help with either external or internal home treatment work. Below is a list of tools we often recommend:

1. The TheraWand: This device was developed especially for internal pelvic floor work. With its curved shape and somewhat pointed tip, the TheraWand can help with trigger point release and the lengthening of too-tight muscles.
2. A foam roller: As mentioned above, foam rollers can be used to both stretch out too-tight muscles and release trigger points.
3. *The Trigger Point Therapy Workbook* by Clair Davies and Amber Davies: A helpful guide for patients who incorporate trigger point release into their home programs.
4. Tennis ball: Tennis balls are a great tool for working on pelvic girdle and trunk muscles.

A note on dilators: we don't recommend them across the board for at-home treatment of pelvic pain. (When we talk about dilators, we're referring to both the vaginal dilators that come in graduated sizes and any of the other handheld devices designed for internal pelvic floor work.) Dilator use is not therapeutic for all cases of pelvic pain and, in fact, can be harmful in some situations. For example, if a woman has vulvar pain that's caused by a dermatologic disease or referred pain from the pudendal nerve, home dilator use could irritate the tissue causing pain while not addressing its underlying cause. So while dilator use would be effective in many situations for male or female patients to treat internal trigger points and/or too-tight muscles, it's important to first ask your PT if it's appropriate in your particular case.

Pain is not gain.

As a general rule of thumb, if any home treatment technique makes a patient feel better, it's a keeper. However, the technique may cause discomfort at the time, typically because impairments exist in the targeted tissue. But if the technique is therapeutic, any discomfort felt in the beginning should dissipate, and symptoms should feel better afterward. If there is soreness afterward and the technique was therapeutic, the soreness will wear off, and the patient will feel better as a result of the treatment. But if the technique escalates pain or symptoms, patients should back off and discuss it with their PT.

Ice or heat?

Ice or heat can be helpful; however, for patients with nerve involvement, ice could exacerbate symptoms, often causing burning pain. If it does, discontinue. If either heat or ice is soothing, continue use.

Use the right lube.

For any type of internal work, a glycerin-free lubricant is the way to go. And if you use medical gloves, we recommend latex-free gloves. That's because both glycerin and latex can be irritating for some.

Do a test run with your PT.

We recommend that a patient test out any technique he/she plans to incorporate into a home treatment program with their PT first to make sure they're doing the technique correctly. For example, if any of our patients will be using a TheraWand or any other tool for internal self-treatment, we have them bring it into PT for a little guidance. What we'll do is actually palpate the muscles the patient is going to be working on at home with the TheraWand, while asking the patient to pay close attention to how the palpation feels. Then we have them do it themselves. After trying out the technique for one week, we ask them at their next appointment how they responded to the treatment and if they have any questions.

"Self-care" at home is just as important as "self-treatment."

Besides all the techniques we discuss above, like internal work and external work, another vital part of a home treatment program is self-care. By this we mean it's important to find certain activities, such as meditation, deep breathing, hot baths, tai chi (or inactivities: restful sleep is a must), that allow you to relax and calm your nervous system. As you've already learned, treating the nervous system is every bit as important as treating a trigger point or connective tissue restrictions.

PELVIC FLOOR DROPS

While every home treatment program should be individualized, every person dealing with pelvic pain can include one therapeutic activity in his/her home program, and we recommend it across the board. We call this exercise the pelvic floor drop. It's now common knowledge that people with pelvic pain usually have too-tight pelvic floor muscles. A pelvic floor drop helps to loosen those tight muscles. Basically, a drop is the opposite of a Kegel. When you do a drop, you're relaxing your pelvic floor. You achieve this relaxation by contracting a few of your pelvic floor's neighboring muscles (in this case your hip flexors, abductors, and external rotators), which in turn dial down the muscle activity of your pelvic floor. When we go through pelvic floor drops with patients during treatment, we initially ask them to lie on their backs with their hips flexed and externally rotated so that their knees are far apart and their feet are together. Basically, when you're in this position, you're doing a deep squat, just on your back, and a deep squat facilitates pelvic floor relaxation. (It's no coincidence that most of the world goes to the bathroom in this position or that a toddler still in diapers does.) Once they're in the desired position, we cue patients to do a pelvic floor drop by asking them to gently relax the area around the anus, as if they were going to pass gas or urinate. We then ask them to hold the position for five seconds on, five seconds off. At first, we have them do this with our finger inserted vaginally or anally in order to determine whether their pelvic floor muscles are achieving a relaxed state. If patients can achieve a drop, we give them positive feedback; if they're doing it incorrectly; we give them cues and/or hints on how to do it correctly. We don't assign patients drops for their home treatment program until they're able to do the exercise correctly in the treatment room. Two other positions help facilitate a drop besides the one described above: a standing deep squat and a child's pose. Both positions also mimic the deep squatting position. Doing a drop in a standing deep squat position has the added benefit of putting gravity and the person's body weight to work while lengthening the pelvic floor muscles. However, not all patients can get into this position because of limitations, such as hip or sacroiliac joint problems, pelvic organ prolapse, or pudendal nerve irritation. For these patients, the "flat back drop" or drops in child's pose are the best way to go. The pelvic floor drop is a first step toward teaching someone both how to relax the pelvic floor and how to regain control of their pelvic floor muscles. Drops can be done several times a day; the more the better! Ultimately we want patients to be able to relax their pelvic floors in any position—not just the three positions mentioned above. Indeed, the great thing about a drop is that it can be done anytime, anywhere. Once you get the hang of it, you can do it sitting at your desk, standing at the stove cooking dinner, or playing with the kids. We once had a patient who said she did them while walking her dog. As a cue, every time her dog would baptize a tree, mailbox, or fire hydrant, she would do a drop. (For instructions on how to do a pelvic floor drop, please click on our YouTube video at https://www.youtube.com/watch?v=K1I4Zu2SLXI.)

TAKE A DEEP BREATH: IT HELPS

Studies have shown that people with pain syndromes are "shallow breathers," meaning they're often in a stressed "fight or flight" state and don't breathe deeply and slowly. Diaphragmatic breathing, also known as "belly breathing," is carried out by contracting the diaphragm, the horizontal muscle between the chest cavity and the stomach cavity. This results in an expansion of the belly rather than the chest. Diaphragmatic breathing has the potential to help pelvic pain for a few reasons. For one thing, the diaphragm works in conjunction with the pelvic floor muscles, so when you inhale during a diaphragmatic breath, the pelvic floor muscles expand, allowing for greater pelvic floor muscle release, relaxation, and blood flow. Try it right now . . . we'll wait. Didn't you feel that nice pelvic floor expansion while you were taking in that big deep breath? This exercise has also been shown to decrease adrenaline and cortisol, two hormones that are often elevated in people with pain and stress. When cuing patients during diaphragmatic breathing, we tell them to place their hand on their belly to make sure it rises and falls with their breath. However, this isn't the only way to approach deep breathing; many safe, effective techniques exist, and we encourage you to find one or more that are a good fit for you.

HOW NOT TO FREAK OUT DURING A FLARE: MOLLY'S STORY

It's. Just. A. Flare. Four little words that pack a lot of power for me, because they instantly put the brakes on an impending panic attack. This wasn't always the case. Used to be that when I'd have a flare-up of my pelvic pain symptoms, it would devastate me, sending me into a panic-filled dark hole. But after some good communication with my PT, and frankly, getting to the other side of a handful of nasty flares, I had an epiphany, one that changed the course of my recovery, and one I'd like to share. As anyone who has gone through the treatment process for pelvic pain can attest to, it can be a complicated journey. No pill, surgery, set number of PT sessions, or any other secret sauce will get you better. What *does* get you better is an interdisciplinary treatment approach, and signing on to be an active member of the team. Throw in a heaping dose of persistence and patience, and that's how you heal from pelvic pain. At any given time, my treatment team has consisted of a pelvic floor PT, a physiatrist (pain management doctor), and a urogy-necologist. Treatments I have had include trigger point injections, Botox injections, epidural injections, nerve blocks, medication, and a home treatment program that included pelvic floor drops and internal pelvic floor muscle stretching with a TheraWand. I consider myself a pelvic pain success story. After a few years of regular PT and working my interdisciplinary treatment plan, I'd say I'm 90% better. Oftentimes, however, healing has felt a lot like taking one step forward and two steps backward. And flares happened. At the beginning they happened A LOT. Even as I write this, I can still recall the feeling of utter despair that would envelop me when I'd have an off-the-pain-scale flare-up. For me, a pain flare meant and continues to mean an intense urethral/ vestibular/vulvar burning coupled with burning sit bone pain and urinary urgency/frequency. A flare would come unexpectedly. I would be having a good day, or a few good weeks, and then *BAM!* I'd feel as though I was back at square one. Sometimes I could connect a specific incident to the flare. A long car trip, sitting for too long, wearing the wrong pants, having sex, traveling, a urinary tract infection; all could set off a three-alarm flare. But other times, a flare would just seemingly come out of nowhere. Whatever was behind the flare, my reaction was always the same: I would hop on the catastrophizing train in my mind. *"All that progress out the window,"* I'd think. *"I'll never get better, I'll never enjoy [insert activity here] again." "My husband is going to leave me." "I'll never be able to have children." "My family and friends are going to abandon me." "I'm going to grow old alone." "Should I ask my doctor if I should try [insert name of drug or type of injection here]?" "I've got to make a plan!!!"* My anxiety would in turn feed the flames of my pain, and up up up my pain levels would go. It wasn't until I began getting regular PT with Stephanie and Liz, who began to educate me about what exactly was causing my symptoms as well as the recovery process, that I was finally able to develop tools that enabled me to stop the train on its tracks. With those tools, I was able to get to the other side of a flare without going into full-scale panic mode. Not only that, but the tools I developed helped me get through a flare *faster*. First, I want to share what I learned about flares: flares may happen as a result of very predictable things, such as a UTI or yeast infection, a bout of food poisoning, overdoing it at the gym, or even repetitive coughing from the flu. It's simply not always possible to avoid a triggering event, even when you know what your triggers are. For instance, stress, travel, and diet are common triggers that are often unavoidable. In addition, when a pain flare can't be tied to any tangible event, the central nervous system can be the culprit. This is because the central nervous system can generate pain without there being tissue damage. I also learned that on occasion a flare is your pelvic floor's way of telling you it's not ready for you to add a particular activity into the mix. For instance, when I began to wear pants again, I realized that there were certain kinds of pants, tight yoga pants for example, that would cause a flare. The pants were the triggering event because my tissues were still impaired. So I gave my cute new yoga pants to my coworker and went back to my looser-fitting yoga pants. Along those same lines, it often happens that as we begin to feel better, we start doing more, and sometimes flares are a reminder to pull back and to slow down. Lastly, it's important to remember that once you reach a level of healing, no matter the intensity of the flare, your body can and will get back to that level. These words of wisdom helped me because I could finally stop feeling as if I had gone backward every time I had a flare—that all the progress I had made had gone out the window. Instead, I realized that the flare was just a temporary bump on the road to recovery, and that made all the difference. It enabled me to keep the alarms in my brain from going off and to calmly take my bag of tools off the shelf and do what I needed to do to take care of myself. This was key for me, because I quickly learned that a negative response to flares could make the flares worse and further aggravate my nervous system. So for me, it was really important to remain calm and relaxed during a flare. "Easier said than done" may be your first response to this advice; however, trusting that my flare was temporary really made an enormous difference in my overall healing process. Since everyone's symptoms are different, what works for me may not be the thing for you. Yet I still want to share the contents of my "flare toolbox" to reflect how you can be proactive in overcoming a flare. I've already mentioned the first trick in my bag, but because it's so effective, it bears mentioning again. I literally take a deep breath and say these words either out loud or in my head: "It's. Just. A. Flare." I wasn't sure why this worked, so I asked Erica Marchand, Ph.D., a licensed psychologist in Los Angeles, to weigh in. "There's some evidence from neuroscience that naming or verbalizing difficult feelings decreases some of their emotional reactivity—'name it to tame it,'" Dr. Marchand explained. "Pain often provokes an automatic emotional reaction, but if we can name it and think about it (what to do about it, what has helped in the past, how long it will last, how to take care of ourselves), it gives us more choice about how to respond." Aside from "naming it to tame it," other tools in my flare toolbox include:

- Ice pack: "Ice." It sounds so simple, and it is, and to this day it still surprises me how effective icing is. It ALWAYS makes me feel better. What I usually do is call it an early night, line up a few of my favorite shows on Netflix or On Demand, and relax in bed with my trusty ice pack (a little chocolate helps too). Typically I'll apply the ice pack to my hot spots for 10 minutes or so. Take a break, repeat, and so on for a few hours until I fall asleep. And voilà! Not only will I feel better in real time, I'll wake up the next day feeling a remarkable improvement in my pain levels, especially my sit bone pain. (I want to acknowledge here that many people with nerve pain can't tolerate ice. These folks benefit more from heat. Also, for many chocolate is a bladder irritant.)
- Stretching: My TheraWand has long been a tool that I've used for self-treatment. When I flare, I find that a gentle stretch with my crystal wand (which I keep in the fridge, so it's always nice and cool) will make me feel better both during the stretching and the following day. I am careful to use an adequate amount of lubrication (which I also keep in the fridge). I find that the cool wand and lubrication help to cool the tissue.
- Medication: As I mentioned above, I have a physiatrist as a member of my treatment team, and she has given me specific medication to take in the event of a flare.

(Again, I want to reiterate that every patient with pelvic pain is different and while these tools work for me, they may not work for everyone. Except for the one below; that one is *universal*.)

- Boundaries: When you deal with a persistent pain issue, one of the things that happens is that you inevitably disappoint your family and friends. We all want to make the people we care about happy. It's part of being human. But when I slip into flare mode, I know from experience that just as important as the ice and the stretching and the medication are rest, relaxation, and keeping my stress levels as low as possible. So I've learned to be okay with turning down invitations or telling my husband that I need to have a quiet, relaxing day/night/weekend. E-mails and telephone calls will inevitably go unanswered, and I've learned to be okay with that, even knowing that the folks on the other end might not be.

CONCLUSION

In this chapter, we've provided some general guidelines to help navigate the at-home self-treatment process. A well-thought-out, individualized home treatment plan has the potential to greatly assist in a patient's recovery. In the next chapter we're going to tackle an issue that can be similarly beneficial—exercise.

10

HOW TO EXERCISE TO STAY FIT WITHOUT FLARING SYMPTOMS

Our patients are typically very active, but when pelvic pain enters the picture, we often find that they'll stop moving altogether for fear of making themselves worse or after reading information online about what they should or shouldn't do. For those who do strive to remain active during recovery, exercising for fitness can cause a flare-up of symptoms, such as urinary urgency/frequency, perineal burning, or vulvar or anal itching, to name a few. Often this happens after patients have taken a break from their fitness routine, either because of their pain or due to that aforementioned fear of making their symptoms worse. When symptoms flare as a result of returning to exercise, patients understandably become frustrated, fearing they'll never be able to get back to the activities they enjoy. Many of our patients are very athletic, and having to stop exercising because of their pain can be devastating. Folks who were once athletes begin to feel "broken" when they can't do an activity seemingly as basic as restorative yoga. We always reassure these patients that it is possible to return to a high level of exercise, in time. And in the meantime, we work with them to put together a plan that allows them to stay active without inducing a flare of their symptoms. Plus, we reassure them that typically if symptoms increase from an activity, it's not because of tissue damage, and that the flare will resolve. Because regular exercise is so important for all-around good health, both physical and emotional, not to mention the proven benefits of exercise on persistent pain (see box below), we want our patients to establish a balance between staying fit and healthy and not exacerbating their symptoms. In doing so, we may need to ask them to modify exercise at first, but always with the goal of getting them back to their desired activities.

After years of working with patients on this issue, and armed with our knowledge of exercise anatomy and physiology, we've compiled a few general exercise tips for those recovering from pelvic pain. But at the end of the day, it's always best to discuss general exercise routines with your PT, who will be in the best position to know exactly what activities will/will not exacerbate your impairments.

GENERAL EXERCISE TIPS

1. Return to exercise slowly.

"When returning to activity, you always want to do more than the day before, but just a little more." This is a quote we borrowed from neuroscientist and pain expert Lorimer Moseley. It embodies in a very practical way the need to return to exercise slowly if you've been inactive for a period of time while in recovery from pelvic pain. Those recovering from pelvic pain are often eager to return to exercise once they're feeling better. Or they get carried away on "good days." We're always excited when patients are eager to return to activity, but we always advise them to temper their excitement with caution. Steady progress should always be the goal. The reason it's important to proceed with caution is that inactivity results in a loss of muscle strength. In addition to having to regain that lost strength, patients often need to regain coordination. To be sure, the coordination between the body and the brain weakens with disuse. Both strength and coordination do come back, but it takes time. So when returning to exercise after a period of inactivity, the best course of action is to scale back on the volume and intensity of whatever workout you did prior to pelvic pain. So if you're a runner who was benched for a bit while recovering from pelvic pain and you used to run 5 miles a day, it might be a good idea to start back at 1 mile a couple of days a week at a slower pace than you're used to, and see how it feels. The longer you've been out of the game, no matter what the exercise, the longer it will take to get back to your previous levels of activity. Another important piece of advice is to listen to your body. Our bodies always tell us when we've done too much.

2. Low-impact cardio is a great place to start.

While recovering from pelvic pain, low-impact cardio is a great activity, as it provides the benefits of getting the heart rate up and the endorphins flowing while not negatively impacting symptoms in the way high-impact activity may. For those with a history of pelvic pain, the best low-impact cardio exercise is walking. For those just starting out, we recommend walking without much of an incline. They can slowly increase their distance every week or so, and once they get to their goal distance, they can work to increase their pace. Then they can work to increase their elevation, but slowly. The key is to find a distance, pace, and incline that does not flare symptoms. If someone was a walker prior to pelvic pain, we tell him/her to start up again at a distance of about one-quarter of what they used to do, but at a slower pace. Once they've reached their goal distance, then they can begin slowly experimenting with pace and elevation. Another good choice for low-impact cardio is walking in water. Because the human body is practically weightless in water, muscles and joints are free of pressure when submerged. For the pelvic floor, this means less pressure bearing down on it as it supports the weight of the body/pelvic organs and maintains posture, so it can relax a bit more than it's used to doing, letting the buoyancy of the water do some of its work. Lastly, for those who like to go to the gym, we recommend the StepMill cardiovascular machine for low-impact cardio. This machine is great because at slower speeds—less than level 5 miles per hour—you get a great cardio workout with the added benefit of strengthening the gluteal muscles.

3. Engage in slower, low-impact exercise when doing strength training.

When getting back to strength training, either after recovering from pelvic pain or during recovery, as a general rule of thumb, slow, low-impact exercises are less likely to cause flare-ups, as they allow for the reprogramming of any faulty movement patterns (recruiting the wrong muscles for a movement) that developed while dealing with pelvic pain. Below are a few examples of these types of exercises:

- Shallow squats: Shallow squats are better because the deeper the squat, the greater the chance faulty movement patterns may creep back in.
- Shallow squats on a foam pad: This movement creates an unstable surface and therefore elicits a beneficial co-contraction of muscles. Plus, it's a safe and effective way to strengthen the gluteal muscles, thighs, and hips.
- Balancing on a Bosu ball or foam roller: If using the Bosu ball, first use the flat side down and progress to the round side down, moving from more stable to less stable.

4. If an exercise begins to hurt, stop.

When returning to exercise during or after recovery from pelvic pain, "no pain, no gain" couldn't be further from the truth! If an activity causes pain, either an increase in pelvic pain symptoms or any other pain, discontinue that exercise. Muscle soreness from a workout is often okay, but pain or an increase in symptoms is not. If you're on the fence about what constitutes "normal" muscle soreness versus pain, discuss it with your PT ASAP. That's his/her area of expertise, and he/she will be able to help you figure it out. Plus, he/she will be able to help you modify the activity or replace it with an entirely new one. All that said, there is one exception where "working through the pain" can be beneficial. That exception is when a patient needs to dial back an amped-up central nervous system. For example, Stephanie had a patient who noticed that using the elliptical machine resulted in symptoms of urinary urgency/frequency and hip pain afterward. After starting PT, the patient learned that a trigger point in her pubococcygeus and a labral tear in her hip were contributing to her symptoms. Although her symptoms improved in PT, the patient was afraid to try the elliptical machine again. When she did work up the nerve to try it, lo and behold, she felt the same discomfort she had prior to PT. She checked in with Stephanie about the matter. Stephanie assured her that her impairments were gone and encouraged her to work through the discomfort, concluding that the patient's central nervous system was at play, and that the fear and anxiety around using the machine were causing her discomfort. The patient took Stephanie's advice and was ultimately able to use the elliptical machine with no symptoms or discomfort.

5. Take care when working out your abdominal muscles.

1. The muscles of the abdominal wall and the pelvic floor are "synergists." This means they assist each other to accomplish movement. For instance, an abdominal muscle contraction will result in a pelvic floor contraction; therefore, some abdominal exercises can exacerbate pelvic pain symptoms if done too early in the recovery process. As a general rule of thumb, people recovering from pelvic pain can work their abdominal muscles once they (a) have no trigger points in any of the muscles activated during the exercise and (b) have regained motor control of their pelvic floor muscles and can relax them after they contract in response to the exercise. Below are the abdominal exercises we recommend to patients with pelvic pain. For a variety of reasons, these exercises typically don't negatively impact the pelvic floor.

- Planks: When you do a plank, pelvic floor activity will increase, but your pelvic floor is not going to contract as much as with a sit-up. Planks are also a better idea than sit-ups because they help to work muscles, specifically the transversus abdominis muscles, that are important in low back and pelvic girdle stability as well as urinary and bowel function. So not only are you doing an exercise that has less of an impact on the pelvic floor, you get more bang for your buck.
- Standing exercises that involve weights on a pulley: When you do these exercises, your abdominal muscles are going to help you remain upright, providing an abdominal workout with less stress on the pelvic floor compared to a sit-up.
- Knee raises sitting on a physio ball: The ball creates an unstable surface, so your abdominal and other pelvic girdle muscles contract to prevent you from falling off. Voilà! Instant workout! Moving the arms or raising the entire leg instead of just the knee can make this exercise harder.

6. Stay away from exercises that increase pelvic floor muscle tone during early symptom onset or early in the recovery process.

Certain exercises will increase pelvic floor tone (tighten muscles), and the majority of impairment-causing symptoms, like too-tight pelvic floor muscles, trigger points, and irritated nerves, can be made worse by increased pelvic floor tone. So these exercises are best avoided for those with a history of pelvic pain. Below is a list of such exercises:

- Activities that involve impact, such as single-leg or double-leg jumping
- Squatting in single-leg stance
- Gym machines versus free weights: Generally speaking, our patients have reported more issues with symptom flare-ups when using machines versus free weights. We theorize that the machines may not be at the proper height or the weights may actually be too heavy for the patient, resulting in more symptoms.
- Deep squats and lunges: When people with pelvic pain do squats or lunges, their hamstrings oftentimes take over instead of their gluteal muscles, which can be detrimental to a tight pelvic floor. Also, those with a history of pelvic pain often have too-tight hip rotators, and this prevents them from doing the exercise properly.
- Biking or spinning: Most people with pelvic pain have problems and pain in the muscles that are compressed on a bike seat, i.e., nearly the entire pelvic floor. So the pressure will aggravate the pelvic floor. In fact, we have had patients whose pain started as a result of biking in the first place. But that's not to say that if you're a passionate cyclist who develops pelvic pain, you'll never be able to ride again. This is definitely a goal we work toward with patients. However, while in recovery from pelvic pain, cycling will likely need to be temporarily put on hold.
- Sitting abduction/adduction machine: Many patients with pelvic pain have trigger points in the muscles these machines target— the inner/outer thighs—so using these machines will often aggravate the trigger points and therefore their symptoms. On top of that, these machines may actually cause pelvic pain and therefore should be avoided.

- Deep squats with heavy weights: Deep squats with heavy resistance are not a good choice. For one thing, it's common for those doing this exercise to recruit the wrong muscles for the movement, thus setting them up for injury. For another thing, this exercise lengthens the pudendal nerve and the pelvic floor muscles, making them both vulnerable to injury. In fact, this activity has actually been known to cause pudendal neuralgia.

ON-THE-FENCE EXERCISES

For some exercises, like biking, it's not hard to understand their potential to negatively impact a pelvic floor in recovery, but there are other, very common exercises, like running for instance, whose effect on a recovering pelvic floor is more nebulous. For these activities, it really does depend on the specifics of the person's case. The good news is that we do have some general guidelines for these workouts.

- Running: For patients who have trigger points in their pelvic girdle muscles or core weakness, running is going to bother their pelvic floor symptoms, but if they are clear in those areas, they can usually slowly get back into running.
- Swimming: Swimming is a great form of exercise. However, certain strokes may be problematic for those who have trigger points in areas that cause pelvic pain. For example, the breaststroke activates the obturator internus muscle, so patients with trigger points in this muscle should choose a different stroke, such as freestyle. Conversely, patients with psoas or hip flexor trigger points may get aggravated symptoms with the freestyle motion but feel comfortable using the breaststroke.
- Pilates and yoga: Yoga and Pilates have a wide range of exercise combinations, and not all are a good fit for a recovering pelvic floor. For example, mat Pilates classes are almost always a bad idea, because sit-ups, aka "100s," are very common in these classes. Certain yoga poses involve a lot of hip flexion, which could exacerbate irritated pelvic floor nerves, specifically the pudendal and posterior femoral cutaneous nerves, which are often involved in pelvic pain. We recommend that with either Pilates or yoga,

PTs and patients work together to figure out if a certain class is a good fit. Read these posts from our blog (http://www.pelvicpainrehab.com/alternative-treatment/815/can-yoga-help-my-pelvic-pain/) for more information on how yoga can be tailored to pelvic floor recovery, and remember timing is everything.

HOW EXERCISE ALTERS HOW WE EXPERIENCE PAIN

Exciting new research shows that regular exercise may alter how a person experiences pain. And the more exercise we do, according to the study, the higher pain tolerance becomes. Scientists have known for a long time that exercise can briefly dull pain. That's because as muscles begin to ache during exercise, our bodies release natural opiates, such as endorphins, that slightly dampen the ache. This is known as exercise-induced hypoalgesia, and it usually starts during the workout and hangs around for about 20 to 30 minutes afterward. But whether exercise can alter the body's response to pain over the long term has remained unclear. Now, thanks to research undertaken at the University of New South Wales in Australia, we're closer to getting an answer. Here's the lowdown: researchers recruited 12 inactive adults who expressed interest in exercising, and another 12 who were similar in age and activity levels but preferred not to exercise. The researchers first tested all the study participants to find out how they reacted to pain. Pain response is extremely individualized and depends on several factors, including pain threshold and pain tolerance. Basically, pain threshold is the point at which someone starts to feel pain, and pain tolerance refers to how much time he/she can put up with the pain before putting a stop to whatever is causing it. Once pain threshold and pain tolerance were noted, the participants were separated into two groups. One group began a program of moderate stationary bicycling for 30 minutes, three times a week, for six weeks. This group progressively became more fit. The other group went about their lives just as they had before signing on to the study. After six weeks, researchers tested the pain thresholds and pain tolerance of all the participants. This is what they found: the participants who did not exercise had no changes in their responses to pain; both their pain tolerance and pain threshold remained the same. As for the participants who exercised, while their pain threshold remained the same, they had a substantial increase in pain tolerance. And the participants who saw the greatest increase in fitness levels had the greatest jump in their pain tolerance. For those who deal with persistent pain, this may mean that moderate amounts of exercise can change their perception of pain, thus helping with daily functioning and leading to a higher quality of life.[1]

Note

1. MD Jones et al., "Aerobic Training Increases Pain Tolerance in Healthy Individuals," *Medicine & Science in Sports & Exercise* 46 (2014): 1640–1647.

TAMRA'S STORY

A Stabbing Pain

I was a busy college freshman only concerned with three things: my studies, tennis practice, and going out swing dancing with my boyfriend. I was young and eager to figure out my place in the world. Every day I would wake up early for tennis practice and hit for a few hours. Then I would quickly wolf down breakfast at the cafeteria and go to my classes before returning in the afternoon for weight lifting, conditioning, and more drills. I was known on the team for my mental toughness and my ability to do whatever it took to win.

That strength would disappear when I first had sharp pain with intercourse the summer after my freshman year. My boyfriend and I had been together for eight months, and up until that point, sex had been pain-free. Obviously concerned, I began seeing several gynecologists. The first told me I had a yeast infection, gave me some medication, and sent me on my way. The pain continued, so I saw another gynecologist on campus who told me I had a UTI, gave me some medication, and sent me on my way. The pain only worsened, and one night during my sophomore year, I felt such a stabbing pain, I found myself in an ambulance on my way to the emergency room. The doctor on call disregarded everything I told him and told me I must have an STD and tried to treat me for it. When I explained this was impossible, as I was in a committed relationship and practiced safe sex, and besides hadn't had intercourse in months, he shook his head and said I must be lying and there was nothing more he could do. I left the ER that night feeling ashamed and misunderstood.

I felt so alone in my pain—no one could see or understand I was hurting. I closed up emotionally for months, unable to tell anyone what I was going through. The pain continued to break me down, and I found it more and more difficult to make it through my schoolwork and daily tennis practices. I began skipping classes because I had difficulty sitting through lectures and placing pressure on my pelvis. If I had to attend class, I brought ice pack pads to put in my underwear and wore bulky sweatpants so no one would know. After continued frustration, I went to a fourth gynecologist, who mentioned vulvar vestibulitis for the first time to me. She explained this was a new diagnosis for women who felt sharp pain around their vulva and referred me to a specialist in Philadelphia for further treatment.

During my first visit to the specialist, I was prescribed an estrogen-based cream to build up the tissue around my vulva. I was also placed on an increasing dosage of an antidepressant as part of a pain control intervention. It had disastrous effects on me. Over the course of the next few months, I experienced extreme emotional swings. I would cry in the shower and found myself yelling at those closest to me. The medication also made me extremely groggy and made it even more difficult to focus on my schoolwork. My dad drove to my school several times a week to type my papers while I would dictate from bed. I no longer felt in control of my body or my mind. It was the furthest from myself that I have ever felt.

Not able to handle the side effects any longer, I returned to my specialist, and I remember sitting across from her in a small, cold room. I was frustrated that my treatments weren't working and wanted answers. She looked into my eyes and told me that vulvar vestibulitis is a chronic condition and that there would always be flare-ups, so I had better prepare myself to live with this for the rest of my life. I felt the last bit of hope in me shatter. I would never get better? How could I continue to live my life like this? The word "chronic" felt like a prison sentence. To me it meant both the certainty that I would have pain and the uncertainty of how it would affect me. I felt trapped. I sat motionless on the train back home that day, watching the world whirl by me. I felt as if my life was rushing past me and I was missing it. To make matters worse, this visit coincided with a bad breakup. We had been together for 2 years, but the weight of my illness became too much for him to handle. I believed no one would ever love me again, that I was cursed to go through this life alone. There was no sense in looking ahead to the future. I was now living day to day.

Since conservative treatment had failed, my specialist signed me up for a vestibulectomy. If the vulva were a clock, this surgery would essentially cut out 4 o'clock to 8 o'clock, the portions that were causing me the most pain, and would replace the tissue with internal vaginal tissue. The issue I had with this last-resort surgery was its narrowed focus. It would cut out the place I first felt pain, but what if there was more to the story? What if my pain came from elsewhere? These were questions I did not have enough knowledge to ask.

It was at this point that I turned to writing and started a health blog called *Sky-Circles* (http://sky-circles.blogspot.com/). The title was based on a poem by Rumi about having hope in the face of struggle. I had always been an avid reader, but I turned to poetry when I was sick—not as a hobby, but as a necessity. I sought solace in the words of Mary Oliver and Rumi. And eventually they inspired me to write. It had been seven long months of misdiagnosis, failed treatments, and continued pain, which I'd kept hidden from everyone but my immediate family. Writing was cathartic and allowed me to share my story. I found a nurturing online community where women could share their experiences and seek guidance. Only weeks before my vestibulectomy, a reader of my blog wrote to me and suggested that I see a women's health physical therapist, because something else could be referring pain to my vulva. She gave me the name of Liz and Stephanie's practice in San Francisco, and after researching what pelvic floor physical therapy entailed, I decided it was time to become proactive about my health. Up until then, I had been allowing my doctors to dictate my plan of care. It was time for me to become educated before making any more medical decisions. I booked an appointment and my flight, and two weeks later, my mom and I found ourselves driving up and down the hills of San Francisco. We would soon learn that up until that point, doctors had been looking at my pain through a narrowed lens. We were about to step back and see the bigger picture.

Finding Answers

It wasn't my first time seeing a women's health physical therapist. I had previously seen two in New Jersey who claimed expertise in the field, but in hindsight, had no idea what they were doing when it came to my case. The first only prescribed Kegel exercises and said I needed to strengthen my pelvic floor. The second used a biofeedback machine to show me I needed to relax my pelvic floor. Going to San Francisco was a completely different experience. Liz performed a comprehensive evaluation that included an internal pelvic and external orthopedic exam. She paid close attention to my hips, testing my flexibility and strength. She also asked extensive questions about my medical and athletic history. At the end of the visit she told me her findings, which included limited range of motion at the hip, indicative of labral tears. She explained that the asymmetrical rotation of tennis led to repetitive motion at the hips, causing stress to the musculature and joint. Liz also explained that hip trauma can refer pain to the pelvic floor. She recommended that I see a sports physician and have imaging done immediately. I flew back to the East Coast feeling more educated and more in control of my future. I was in the middle of my junior year and felt hopeful for the first time that I would make it to graduation pain-free.

Sure enough, I had tears in both my left and right labrum and spent the next two summers getting them repaired. They ended up being two of the biggest tears my surgeon had ever seen and required extensive rehabilitation. I found a new pelvic floor physical therapist in NYC, who did extensive internal and external manual physical therapy work. In addition, she worked to strengthen and stretch my hips. We discovered my pelvic floor was extremely tight, as well as my obturator internus and piriformis muscles. This explained why sitting had been so painful. Slowly I started improving and feeling more like myself. My hips became stronger, and I felt ready to get back to my life. When I became a senior, I was named captain of my university's tennis team. I put my patient identity to the side and became an athlete again. I played my heart out, but as the matches continued, the pain in my hips returned. I had to stop playing halfway through the year to focus more on my recovery.

Although my hip surgeries were successful, I was still having set-backs in my treatment. I continued to have pain throughout my body. I found a new pelvic health specialist and went through two years of Traumeel injections, a natural anti-inflammatory to help reduce pain. She would give them to me at certain trigger points around my vulva, vaginal opening, gluteal muscles, and hips. The injections only lasted a few minutes, but needle injections into your vagina and deep into your muscles is not an easy procedure to sit through. I would have to bring a pad for the walk home to prevent the blood from staining my under-wear.

Around this time I finished my degree and accepted an exciting opportunity to work in environmental advocacy in Denver. I wasn't healthy yet, but I was tired of waiting to start my life. In many ways, I needed an escape. Unfortunately, after less than two months of work-ing, I called home in tears and explained to my parents that I couldn't do it anymore. My parents, steadfast in their love and support, picked me up from the airport that weekend.

Back home with my parents, I went through yet another surgery, repairing tears along my pubic bone and surgically releasing my tight adductor muscles. I was infuriated and upset that yet again, my life was back on hold. I was still having difficulty sitting for longer than 15 minutes and dealt with constant, unshakable pain. But giving up wasn't an option for me. I went to physical therapy after my third surgery and was referred to a pain doctor for prolotherapy injections. These differed from my previous injections because they were more aggressive and required longer sessions.

Every month for the next year I went through trigger point injec-tions in my hip, pelvic, and gluteal regions, the idea being that the irritant glucose solution would trigger the body's natural healing pro-cess and repair damaged areas. Each treatment was over an hour of repetitive injections with long needles. Out of all the things I went through, these treatments were undoubtedly the worst. During the first one, I was unprepared but managed to stay silent until I curled up in the back of the car while my mom drove me home. I cried and cried and cried. I cried out in pain, for going through something so awful, for not knowing when it would end. I cried because I wanted to be braver, stronger, better. I cried because it felt right and because I needed it and because I wanted to feel something other than pain.

And so, having been there myself, I want to tell you that it is okay to be at your worst. To cry your heart out because you feel defeated and alone and scared. It's okay to feel pain, to lose control and run away for a while. It's okay to lean on your friends and family. It's okay to be vulnerable and ask for help and see a therapist. It's okay to shut yourself down and lock yourself in your room. Just do whatever you can to make it through the day. Know that change is the only constant in life, and tomorrow always brings new possibilities. After six months of enduring the difficult prolotherapy treatments, I finally started to notice a decrease in my pain.

A New Calling

I continued to document my medical and emotional struggles online, since writing was so therapeutic. My blog began to grow in readership as more women searched for answers. It soon reached tens of thousands of readers from across the world. What had begun as a personal release became an avenue to spread awareness about an unknown and too-often-misunderstood topic. I unexpectedly became a confidant and mentor to others struggling with pelvic pain. I even appeared on an MTV *True Life* episode to further advocate for pelvic floor health, especially the intimate connection between the hips and pelvis. I received hundreds of e-mails from readers expressing their gratitude for my openness and asking for help in their own medical struggles. As I read more of these e-mails, I realized I could offer more than just an encouraging response or a referral. One day I was sitting in the exam chair at my specialist's office and suddenly realized that I should become a women's health physical therapist. Despite the barriers of going back to school and my continuing health problems, I wanted to help others find answers sooner than I had found mine. I wanted to offer comprehensive medical care that looked at the whole body, the whole person. I wanted to help others overcome struggle and hardships and help them persevere and make a meaningful life for themselves. And so I set off to give my own life more meaning.

In August 2012, I started at Thomas Jefferson University in Philadelphia. Since then, I have worked toward my doctorate degree in physical therapy and my dream of becoming a pelvic floor physical therapist. As I find myself mere months from graduation, I am excited and eager to begin and help my patients heal. My dream is to develop a practice that emphasizes holistic pelvic health, with a focus on female athletes. I want to develop protocols for this demographic to prevent injuries like mine from befalling others.

While working toward that goal, I've been able to focus on my health as well as my schoolwork. During the first year of my studies, I worked with a new pelvic floor PT in Philadelphia to manage my residual pain through aggressive manual work, strengthening exercises, and stretching. I'm happy to report that after that first year I've not been back to PT and have stopped all injection treatments. I've also fallen in love and now have pain-free sex for the first time in years. Plus, I'm beginning to love my body instead of seeing it as a battleground. I continue to live pain-free through preventive care, such as maintaining a healthy, balanced diet, stretching tight musculature, training with functional movement, strengthening my core and pelvic floor, and practicing healthy body mechanics. I also focus on emotional health, reducing stressors in my life with meditation, reading, and yoga.

People often ask what helped me the most during my recovery. With such a complicated medical history and trying so many different interventions simultaneously, it's difficult to pinpoint the exact medical impetus for my healing. After going through physical therapy school, I firmly believe in the strong connection between the pelvic floor and the hips. The surgeries I went through fixed my body's mechanical problems, while the proceeding physical therapy strengthened muscles that were weak and stretched muscles that were overcompensating. The most useful thing for me during this entire process was the attainment of knowledge. Self-education allowed me to take control over my own health care. As a physical therapist, it's a requirement to be a lifelong learner, but I urge everyone to actively seek information so that they can be proactive about their health.

Stronger than Ever

What began as a sharp, localized pain in June 2007 grew to encompass a mind-body seven-year journey. As I write this, I'm currently in the best physical shape of my life, even better than my years as a collegiate athlete. I go to the gym daily and especially love serious weight lifting. I have climbed Kilimanjaro, the tallest mountain in Africa, along with several other high mountain peaks in the United States. And on my 26th birthday, I ran my first marathon. It was a long journey, full of ups and downs. When I was in the midst of my pain, I would have done anything for someone to take it away from me. When I felt the most broken, a dear friend gave me a small Japanese pot with several gold lines. I thought it was an unusual gift until I read the card, which said it was a piece of Kintsugi pottery. It's a Japanese method of fixing cracked pottery with gold or silver and represents more than an art form. It's also a philosophy of life. The Japanese believe there is beauty in being broken, that cracks should be celebrated and not concealed. They also believe the gold fillings reinforce the pottery, making it stronger than it was before.

About Tamra: Tamra Wroblesky graduated from Thomas Jefferson University with a doctorate in physical therapy in 2015 and is currently focused on building her pelvic floor physical therapy practice in New Jersey. Prior to moving her pelvic pain advocacy to the treatment room, Tamra shared her experiences recovering from pelvic pain on her blog titled *Sky-Circles*. In addition, her pelvic pain story has been featured on MTV's mini-documentary show, *True Life*.

CONCLUSION

In this chapter we've offered guidelines intended to help those dealing with pelvic pain stay fit without flaring their symptoms. For so many reasons staying fit is important for those recovering from pelvic pain. But we know how tough it can be for a formerly active person to be faced with the pelvic pain recovery process. However, often they channel the drive and motivation they've acquired in sportsmanship to the task. Another challenge that those with pelvic pain face can be communicating with providers, especially when a team of providers from different specialties is involved in their treatment. This is the topic we cover in the next chapter.

11

TIPS FOR OPTIMIZING COMMUNICATION WITH YOUR PROVIDERS

For five years Kylee has been dealing with endometriosis. For the past year, her symptoms of abdominal, vaginal, and low back pain have gotten much worse. They've gone from intermittent pain just before and during her menstrual cycle to constant, 24/7 pain that has begun to interfere with her daily life. Believing that her pelvic floor muscles were most likely behind Kylee's uptick in symptoms as opposed to the disease process of her endometriosis, Kylee's doctor referred her to PT. And indeed, Kylee's PT found several impairments she believed to be the culprits behind Kylee's symptoms. Kylee made steady progress in PT, but after a few months, her PT suggested she try trigger point injections as a complementary treatment approach. The PT referred Kylee to a local physician for the injections. The trigger point injections were helpful, and Kylee was pleased with the way her treatment was progressing. It was wonderful to have so many nonsurgical options available to treat her symptoms. At the same time, however, she felt a bit overwhelmed having to juggle so many different providers. Not only was she seeing her PT weekly as well as the new physician for biweekly trigger point injections, she was also still under the care of the physician who had treated her endometriosis for the past five years, a pain management doctor, and an acupuncturist. She found herself struggling to keep everything straight with her different providers, not only in her own mind, but also between her treatment team. For example, she often had a hard time explaining what was happening in PT to her physicians. Kylee was motivated to do everything necessary to get better, and her gut told her that keeping all of her medical providers on the same page would help her reach her treatment goals sooner. But seeing multiple providers for one medical condition was new terrain for her, and she wasn't quite sure what steps were appropriate for her to take to ensure that she and her medical providers were all on the same page.

Kylee's experience is not unique. Many people with pelvic pain find themselves in a position where they have to work to coordinate care between multiple medical providers. The provider-patient relationship itself already comes fraught with its own communication challenges, especially in today's managed care environment where so many providers are pressed for time. Is it any wonder that patients can become overwhelmed? That's why we've decided to dedicate this chapter to providing advice to patients on how to best optimize communication—not only between themselves and their providers, but also between the providers who make up their interdisciplinary treatment team. We'll begin the chapter with some general tips for how patients can improve communication with each of their individual providers. Then we'll share advice on how they can best optimize communication with their PTs. Lastly, we'll reveal a few strategies patients can use to make sure their treatment team members are all on the same page.

TIPS FOR COMMUNICATING WITH PROVIDERS

Be proactive.

As you know by now, pelvic pain is a multilayered condition that crosses medical disciplines. In other words, it can be complicated. As you've also learned, there is no silver-bullet treatment for pelvic pain. It's simply not a condition where a doctor can "fix" the patient or where any one medical provider is likely to have all the answers. So patients have to be active participants in their treatment—a passive approach is just not going to cut it. What does this mean in the context of provider-patient communication? For one thing, it means that when you're at your appointment with your provider, make sure you're actively involved in the discourse. Ask questions if you don't fully understand what your provider is saying. And if you process information better by reading it, feel free to ask your provider if he/she has any articles or other written information you can take home with you or if he/she can recommend any resources for you to check out. Also, don't be afraid to suggest treatment options to your providers based on your own research. Some patients may feel it's not their place to suggest treatment options. Rest assured, living in the Internet age, where so much information is available to patients, means medical providers understand that patients are better informed today than ever before. Therefore, at this point, they're used to patients suggesting options for treatment. But here's a tip nonetheless: a great way to approach any provider about whether a particular treatment option might be worth trying out is to bring in research on the treatment. If you do this, you're speaking the language of your medical providers, and chances are they'll be more comfortable trying something new that they hadn't thought of themselves.

Be prepared.

The majority of medical providers, physicians especially, are overloaded with patients, and their time with you is limited. So to maximize the time you have with them, be extra prepared for your appointments. For example, arrive at your first appointment with any provider with a concise history of your symptoms. It's a good idea to write it down beforehand complete with any pertinent dates, such as when you had a particular surgery or other intervention. Also, for each successive appointment, take some time, even if it's on the drive to the office, to prepare your thoughts beforehand. You know your provider will ask you how your symptoms have been since the last time he/she saw you. So be sure and have your response to this question ready to go. And be as specific as possible about your symptoms. If your pain increased, be specific about exactly what symptom worsened, exactly how it feels, and where the pain is located. The same goes for any interventions you may have tried since the last time you saw a provider. Explain exactly what your reaction was to the intervention, whether it was medication, injections, or even your first round of PT appointments. And also have any questions for the provider at the ready. Again, jot them down if it helps you remember. Lastly, if you communicate with your provider via e-mail, make sure any e-mails you send are clear and concise, and instead of sending several e-mails, try your best to limit the number of e-mails you send.

Be honest.

It's human nature for patients to want to please their medical providers. But it's important that you're always completely honest with them. For example, never minimize your symptoms for fear of disappointing a provider. You won't hurt his/her feelings if a particular treatment didn't work (or even flared your symptoms). The provider's goal is to help you get better, and in order to do this, he/she needs all the information you can give him/her about your condition. If you think about it, medical providers who treat a persistent pain condition rely heavily on what patients tell them. There simply aren't barrages of tests they can do to determine how a patient's treatment is progressing. For that reason, what you report to your providers is key to allowing them to give you the best care possible. So be honest with them, even if that means telling them your symptoms haven't improved since the last time you saw them or that you actually feel worse. It's also human nature for patients to want to present themselves in the best possible light to their providers for fear of being judged. But again, a provider must have an accurate picture of your condition in order to make the best decisions possible for your treatment. So for example, if your PT prescribed a home exercise program for you to do between appointments, and you didn't do it for whatever reason, be honest about it. That way, the PT won't think that the therapeutic exercises simply were not helpful. Also, some people with pelvic pain are embarrassed to share certain details with their providers that are relevant to their recovery—details about their urinary, bowel, or sexual function. This is understandable, but again, it's vital for providers to have all the facts of your case in order to make the best decisions possible. So if you're one of these folks, remind yourself that most medical providers have heard it all, and the details you find embarrassing are likely pretty run-of-the-mill for the provider.

OPTIMIZING COMMUNICATION WITH YOUR PT

When we're evaluating or treating patients, we're constantly explaining to them what we're doing and why. On top of explanations throughout the appointment, at the end of every appointment we give our patients a brief verbal summary of what we did, what we found, and what our expectations are for the progression of their recovery. While it's the job of a PT to keep patients in the loop about the therapeutic techniques they're using during PT, for a variety of different reasons, patients may not get all the information they need to fully grasp what's going on with their treatment. Plus, the dynamic between PT and patient can sometimes be tricky. Oftentimes patients are hesitant to question their PTs for fear of insulting them or disrespecting their expertise. Therefore, they may feel too intimidated to speak up when they have questions or concerns about their treatment. This lack of communication can be detrimental to pelvic floor PT for many reasons, not the least of which is that for some patients, successful treatment will require a major time and emotional commitment. So if a patient is confused or frustrated about treatment, he/she might ultimately decide to throw in the towel and discontinue PT, even though in the long run it's the best treatment option for them. For another thing, a full understanding of the treatment process results in less anxiety. And remember, when anxiety levels go down, it's possible for pain levels to follow suit. Therefore, when it comes to PT for pelvic pain, it's vital that patients be kept in the loop. So at any time during the process, if you as a patient have a question or concern, don't hesitate to bring it up with your PT. He/she wants you to be an active member of your treatment team and will welcome your desire to understand what's going on. Another important area of communication between patient and PT involves patient feedback. Patients must be sure that during their treatment they are providing their PTs with necessary and important feedback. For example, if what the PT is doing is providing relief, it's important that the patient communicate that to the PT. Conversely, if treatment is causing increased pain, it's important for patients to speak up and to describe in as much detail as possible exactly what they're experiencing. This type of feedback helps PTs evaluate their patient's progress and helps them determine if they need to make any treatment adjustments. Lastly, it's important that patients inform their PT of any relevant occurrences between appointments and that they answer their PT's questions to the best of their ability. Again, this information enables the PT to evaluate and modify his/her treatment approach throughout the treatment process. A good tip for making sure you remember exactly how you responded to treatment is to jot down a quick note one, two, or even three days after treatment. That way, when you see your PT again after an entire week has gone by, you'll have those notes to help you recall details you otherwise might forget.

It's important to understand that the information you need to communicate with your PT will change as you progress in treatment. To be sure, you'll want to discuss certain topics with him/her at the beginning of PT, when you reach mid-treatment, and then when it comes time for you to be discharged. For example, at the beginning of treatment, ask your PT what his/her findings were, how the impairments he/she found are causing your symptoms, and what he/she plans to do to try and resolve those symptoms. Then mid-treatment, it's a good idea to ask him/her how you're progressing and if there is anything you should be doing to expedite your treatment. Upon discharge, good questions to ask are how you can maintain the gains you've made in PT and what, if any, signs you should look for if you have to come in for a tune-up. For instance, should you come in if you have a one-day relapse of symptoms, or should you wait until you've had a few symptom relapses before calling to make an appointment?

TIPS FOR KEEPING YOUR INTERDISCIPLINARY TEAM ON THE SAME PAGE

- Pick the member of your treatment team you're the most comfortable with and ask him/her if they are willing to take a leadership role in your case and to act as a facilitator. As we've said in earlier chapters, this provider will often be the PT simply because he/she spends the most time with the patient and he/she is dealing with the neuromuscular system, which is so often a main driver of pelvic pain. However, other providers may be willing to take on this role as well. The patient will have the best sense of which member of his/her team is the best fit for the job.

- Ask providers to write down any technical information you need to update the other providers on your team. For instance, Liz had a patient who was receiving regular trigger point injections from a physician. Because it was hard for the patient to remember the names of the different muscles where Liz found trigger points that might benefit from injections, he had her write them down on a sticky note at each appointment. He asked the doctor to do the same each time he injected the muscles.
- Ask providers to send a copy of their notes to other providers. When we evaluate a patient for the first time, we write up an evaluation summary. In the summary we include a list of our objective findings along with our assessment and treatment plan. We repeat this exercise several times along the way as we reassess patients, and in each instance, we send these treatment summaries to the other providers on the patient's treatment team. This way, the necessary providers are kept abreast of exactly how patients are progressing in PT.
- Ask a provider to give another provider a call to talk. In our role as PTs, we often call other providers to confer on a patient. For example, if we come across a contributing factor that falls under the bailiwick of the provider or if we have an idea for treatment that the provider can carry out, such as administering injections or adding a certain medication to the patient's treatment plan, we simply give him/her a call to discuss it.
- If you gauge that your provider may be interested, ask him/her if he/she would be interested in co-treating you with another provider. For example, we've had many instances in our practice where physicians, other PTs, and/or acupuncturists have come to our clinic to co-treat a patient in order to collaborate in person about his/her treatment. This is beneficial because it allows both providers to evaluate the patient at the same time, giving each insight into how the other examines the patient. For instance, we've found it helpful to hear the questions that other providers ask our patients as well as the patients' responses. This gives us invaluable insight into how the other provider assesses the patient. Gaining this level of understanding of another component of a patient's treatment plan can help providers fine-tune their own treatment strategy. Additionally, if two providers get the opportunity to work on a particular impairment together during an appointment, the hope is that the impairment will be more success-

fully treated. For example, if the patient has a trigger point in one of her hip muscles that the PT thinks would benefit from dry needling, but the patient's acupuncturist is having problems locating the trigger point, the PT can provide guidance as to where to place the needle.

In this chapter we've given patients some tips we believe will enable them to better navigate an interdisciplinary treatment plan, which many folks dealing with pelvic pain have little to no experience with. In fact, so many people in the midst of recovering from pelvic pain have never been in a situation where they've had to focus so many resources— mental, emotional, financial, the list goes on—on their recovery. That's why in the next chapter, we offer some tips for navigating day-to-day living while in recovery for pelvic pain.

12

TIPS FOR DAY-TO-DAY LIVING

In this book, we've covered at length all the different treatment options available for pelvic pain, but so often, recovery from a persistent pain condition isn't just about what goes on in a doctor's office or in the PT treatment room; it also involves a great deal of day-to-day self-care. When we talk about day-to-day self-care, we're talking about the everyday measures folks take to further their recovery. And that's what this chapter is about. In it, we'll discuss a few general self-care tips that we frequently pass along to patients. In addition, we include some tried-and-true tips in the words of former patients. Lastly, because it's not just normal, day-to-day living that can pose challenges to patients, we're going to wrap up the chapter with a discussion of how to survive the holidays, advice that can be easily applied to any special occasion.

A FEW TIPS FOR DAY-TO-DAY LIVING

Cushions

For many who are in recovery from pelvic pain, sitting is a pain trigger. For that reason, we often have to help patients develop strategies that will make sitting more tolerable. Using a cushion when sitting can be helpful. When shopping for a cushion in the marketplace, we advise patients to look for one that will provide pressure relief to the areas that are painful for them when they sit, such as the perineum, tailbone, or vulva, or cushions that distribute their weight more evenly when they sit, thus reducing pressure on certain areas of the pelvis, such as the sit bones or tailbone. But at the end of the day, the best cushion is the one that makes sitting the most comfortable. Our patients have used a handful of commercially available cushions in the past, such as the Thera-Seat (http://www.theraseat.com/) cushion. Two other companies, Cushion Your Assets (www.cushionyourassets.com) and WonderGel (https://wondergel.com/), manufacture cushions that might be helpful to those in recovery from pelvic pain. Sometimes, however, finding the right cushion takes a bit of creativity. For instance, we've had patients who have used padded or gel-covered medical toilet seat covers as cushions, often covering them with homemade slipcovers. Patients have also reported success using more than one type of cushion throughout the day—for example, they might use a different cushion in the car versus when sitting at a desk. Also, replacing a desk chair with a physio ball has been helpful for some of our patients. Unfortunately, finding the "right" cushion for you may turn out to be a lengthy and expensive endeavor. To be sure, we've had patients who've had to keep trying (and buying) cushions until they found the one that worked best for them. However, our thinking is that if your pain increases with sitting and your daily routine involves a lot of sitting (long commute in the car, sitting at a desk), it's worth investing the time and money in finding the right cushion for you.

Clothing

For some patients, clothing is a pain trigger. For example, many women with vulvar pain can't wear jeans or pants because they find the inseam irritating. Some of our patients have found that wearing jeans can be made tolerable if they use a product called the Go Commandos patch (http://www.gocommandos.com/), an adhesive underwear alternative that will cover the inseam. In general, if clothing is a trigger, we advise patients to wear loose clothing that doesn't put pressure on painful areas. For our female patients this often means forgoing underwear, jeans, and pants until they feel better and opting for skirts and dresses instead. And for our male patients, this typically means wearing no underwear and baggier pants and/or shorts with lower inseams.

Shoes

Because so many people with pelvic pain have pain with sitting, they end up standing a great deal longer day in and day out than the average person. For this reason alone, wearing supportive footwear is important to minimize fatigue and/or discomfort in the back, feet, and/or legs when standing. Wearing supportive footwear could mean simply wearing good, supportive sneakers or it could mean using shoe inserts. Patients often ask us if store-bought shoe inserts are sufficient or if custom orthotics are necessary. There is no cut-and-dried answer to this question. Typically we tell patients to start with inexpensive, store-bought orthotics and to use them on a trial basis to see if they are comfortable and lessen lower body fatigue and/or discomfort. If they don't do the trick, then we refer them to a trusted podiatrist for custom-fitted orthotics. Another bit of advice regarding shoes is that flip-flops and high heels should be worn only on rare occasions! That's because for their part, flip-flops do not provide arch support, which can be detrimental from a musculoskeletal perspective. And heels change a person's center of gravity in a way that puts pressure on the low back and pelvic floor. As with many things concerning treatment for pelvic pain, consulting your PT about what sort of footwear is best for your particular situation is always the best way to go.

LIFE HACKS FROM PATIENTS

When we talk to patients recovering from pelvic pain about challenges they face in their everyday lives, the discussion inevitably turns to three topics: communicating an "invisible" condition to family and friends; finding a helpful support system; and the challenge of setting limits with others. Below is some wise advice from folks who have faced these challenges head-on.

A PAIN TO EXPLAIN: CORA'S STORY

In December 2006 my life came to a butt-numbing, crotch-burning halt. My husband and I were on a flight to California. Halfway through the flight, I started to go numb in the "down there" region. I squirmed in my seat in fear, praying that we were close to landing. I leaned over and whispered to my husband that I was losing feeling in my crotch and thighs. Being an emergency medicine doctor, he went straight into ER mode. He thought I might be having a spinal cord emergency and that as soon as we landed, we may need to get to a hospital for a stat MRI scan. Although I made it through that weekend without an ER visit, a few weeks later I had another episode, which in the famous words of my husband "bought me a ticket to the ER." At the hospital, I learned I had injured some delicate muscles I didn't even know I had, and apparently one of my nerves was a little ticked off too. The more formal diagnoses: pelvic floor dysfunction (PFD) with pudendal neuralgia (PN). Ah, such a clinical name for "pain in the ass." I later learned that *pudendal* is the Latin word for "shame." "Great," I thought, "I have a shameful, painful condition. How do I explain that?" It didn't take long for family and friends to hear that I had an injury and was in bed on pain medication. Lots of pain medication. I called my dog-training students and canceled sessions and made arrangements to have the house cleaned and the farm chores done. Like it or not, I was down for the count and closed for business. When family and friends suddenly see an active, healthy woman flat in bed and unable to sit, they ask questions. "What did you do, exactly?" "Can it be fixed?" "Why can't you sit?" What hurts?" "How could this happen to you? You're so healthy!" The questions were endless. How you choose to respond to such questions is a very personal decision. I found with some family members, there was the "too much information" factor. For instance, for my older brother, just hearing "back pain" was plenty. Then there are the old soul friends with whom I was able to share many details. With them I've been able to talk about the dark, scary, sleepless nights. I've whined about the lack of sex in my marriage. I've also shared with them the private details of PT and the more humorous spin I tend to put on this whole deal. When thinking about whom you tell and what you tell them, it is important to think about the motivation of the person asking. Is this a close friend with genuine concern? Is this person a snoopy neighbor or colleague? Is this person really a friend? I've given all sorts of responses, and some have been more tactful than others. I remember one male acquaintance who kept asking for more details. Finally I said to him, "If I tell you any more details, I'm certain you'll blush!" He never asked me another question again. For a while I was telling people that I have a back injury with some muscle and nerve trauma. But that explanation was met with numerous recommendations about back cures, which became tiresome. Now I am more relaxed about the whole thing. If someone asks me, I give a brief and vague response. This usually happens when I am in a public place and some chivalrous man will offer me his seat. Really, they still do that! I politely reject the offer, and if they persist, I say, "Thanks, I'm more comfortable standing. I have an injury." My PT gave me some incredible advice. I asked her how to respond to inquiries regarding my sudden need to stand up all the time and all the other lifestyle changes that accompany the spectrum of PFD. She said that I might ask, "What is it that you'd like to know?" I love that response. It allows for a gentle pause, and time for the other person to respectfully reframe their question or change the subject. I don't think there are any easy ways to communicate what PFD truly is to others in our everyday lives. Even our doctors and PTs have trouble at times. What I think is most important is that as we work toward healing, we do our best to surround ourselves with a caring support system. I have shed many tears in my horse's fur on a quiet night in the barn. And ya know, he never asked "Why?"

SETTING UP A SUPPORT SYSTEM

Cora's Story

Pelvic pain is not something we run marathons for or distribute ribbons for. On the contrary, it's an invisible condition, and for that reason, those dealing with it can feel isolated and alone at a time when they need support more than ever. One of the things I did to make sure I had a strong support system in place during my recovery is I began seeing a therapist. I wanted to maintain as much normalcy as possible, but I knew I needed someplace to vent, and I discovered early on that talking to family worried them, and I didn't want to worry them. Plus I knew they didn't get it. Seeing a therapist provided me with a safe outlet where I could unload. It was so helpful to know I had a standing appointment each week with someone who would help me work through the many ups and downs that come along with a persistent pain condition.

Justin's Story

The best support I got was from another guy around my own age who also had pelvic pain. My therapist put me in touch with him. He was a high-powered lawyer, and it was really encouraging for me to meet someone who had been through what I was going through. It made me feel less isolated. Also, I got some amazing advice from him, which helped me to change my attitude about my own situation. For one thing, he stressed how important it was for me to comply with treatment. It was inspiring to me to see how he worked PT and his home treatment plan into his busy schedule. For another thing, he helped me to realize that during recovery, flare-ups happened, and that they were only temporary setbacks. He said when he would have a flare, instead of giving in to depression and discouragement, he would simply view them as a reminder to continue to be vigilant about his treatment plan. But perhaps most important of all, he was integral in helping me realize that while I was in recovery, I still needed to live my life. For instance, he swam, and maybe that was a little painful, but it was better than being inactive. Also, he'd go out to dinner, and maybe sitting would cause him discomfort, but the social interaction was worth it.

SETTING LIMITS

Georgia's Story

Going through life, it's normal to want to please others. It's just human nature. But when you have to deal with a persistent pain condition (or any major health issue for that matter), your well-being has to become your priority. And a major part of focusing on your own well-being is to learn to set limits and to say, "No, I'm sorry, but I can't." This is not always easy. Pelvic pain is an invisible condition, and so often those who are dealing with it look perfectly healthy and robust. Therefore, the people in their lives struggle to understand why they can't make firm plans or keep commitments. When my pain first started and I found myself having to turn down invitations or when I simply couldn't show up for the people in my life in all the ways I had before, I spent a lot of time stressing myself out about it or even worse, pushing myself to do things that hindered my recovery for fear of disappointing others. Eventually I began to realize that setting limits was an important part of taking care of myself, and that by working so hard to not let others down, I was ultimately letting myself down. A couple of things helped me deal with the repercussions that sometimes came along with setting limits and boundaries with the people in my life. For one thing, I realized (with the help of a therapist) that disappointment is a part of life and that I needed to be okay with disappointing others in situations where my intention was to take care of my health. Second (again with the help of a therapist), I realized that by setting limits and taking care of myself I was actually taking care of the people in my life who depended on me, my husband and son. This resonated with me, because like so many people dealing with pelvic pain, it was important to me that I continue to be there for my family. Reframing limit setting as taking care of my family as well as myself really helped put things into perspective for me, allowing me get past a lot of unnecessary guilt and anxiety.

PELVIC PAIN HOLIDAY SURVIVAL GUIDE: MOLLY'S STORY

"It's the most wonderful DREADFUL time of the year!" A few years ago, that's how I felt about the holidays. It was not always thus. Used to be I was the holidays' biggest fan. As soon as the Halloween candy hit the grocery store shelves, I'd feel a pang of excitement that lasted right up until my hangover on New Year's Day. Turkey. Stuffing. Green bean casserole. Gaudy Christmas lights. Johnny Mathis's velvety voice on the radio. Watching *A Christmas Story* on a loop. Frenzied Christmas shopping! Presents! Christmas cookies! I loved it all! But when I began dealing with a persistent pelvic pain issue, my holiday joy turned to holiday dread. At the first whiff of Halloween candy a cloud of anxiety would settle over me. What was once a thrilling time of the year became a time of stress, frustration, disappointment, and resentment. Not to mention jacked-up pain levels. The good news is that with some trial and error, I've come to once again embrace the holiday season. In fact, my holiday love affair is stronger than ever now *because* of all the lessons I was forced to learn. Before I get into how I learned to embrace the holiday season again, let me first explain my reasons for souring on it to begin with. Managing a chronic pain condition forces you to take care of yourself. Toward that end, my regimen included weekly PT sessions, taking my meds on time, self-treatment, frequent icing, wearing clothes that didn't irritate my hot spots (living in Southern California meant I could wear comfy skirts and dresses practically year-round), getting enough rest and exercise, and eating well. Once the holidays rolled around, much of that went out the window. For me, the holidays required travel and prolonged family visitation. For both Thanksgiving and Christmas my husband and I would spend a week or so with either his family or mine. And while it was wonderful to be among family, the travel, having to veer off my self-care routine, and the marathon socializing was tough, and not only caused my pain to flare, but a great deal of anxiety to boot, which exacerbated the flare.

Turns out I was not alone. "A lot of people with chronic pain go into the holidays with free-floating anxiety on how it's going to go," said Dr. Erica Marchand, Ph.D. and licensed psychologist. "So it colors the whole experience." Dr. Marchand asks her patients who are in this predicament to pinpoint the things they're worried about the most. "Because it's usually not everything, even though it feels like everything." Once patients pinpoint the things they're most worried about, she helps them develop "survival strategies" for getting past their anxiety. In addition to asking patients to pick out what they're most worried about, she asks them to name the things they're looking forward to most. "Realize that these are the activities you really want to do, so that if need be, you can cancel or not accept other invitations. That way you'll have the energy to feel good enough to do the things that lift you up during the holiday season. Because it's not just about making your family happy, it's also about enjoying yourself." For my part, when I sat down to really figure out what it was about the holiday season that I dreaded most, I realized it was the pressure to be the perfect wife, daughter, daughter-in-law, aunt, sister, friend, etc. I hate disappointing people, and during the holidays, especially during family visits, there were a lot more people to potentially disappoint. For example, If I was in too much pain or too tired to join in on some activity or needed some time alone to ice after a long day of sitting and wearing not-so-comfortable clothes (sundresses don't fly everywhere in December), family and friends didn't always get it. "Often we set perfectionist standards for ourselves," said Dr. Marchand. "I think it's important to realize this and to then cut ourselves some slack. You just need to be a *good enough* wife, daughter, mom, sister, friend." "Not to mention," she added, "that usually we ourselves think about our perceived shortcomings so much more than whomever we're worried we've offended. So I think it's important to ask 'Am I allowing myself to feel too guilty about this? Am I allowing a family member/friend to make me feel too bad about this? Is it perhaps okay that I had to cancel plans, and that someone is disappointed because of it?'" And to remember that everybody cancels plans sometimes, and not everyone always feels well. For me, once I realized this—that it was okay if someone was disappointed, and that typically they'd just process it, get over it, and still love me at the other end—it was a life changer. I realized I didn't have to manage everyone's reactions or emotional responses.

That led me to understand that I myself had my own issues with being disappointed with my family and friends around the holiday season. I realized that when I thought they weren't being understanding enough about my limitations, I became resentful, and nothing can dampen holiday cheer like good old-fashioned resentment! It was then that I realized that I myself had to be more empathetic. It occurred to me that it is extremely difficult to really *get* what someone dealing with persistent pain is going through. "It's an invisible condition," explained Dr. Marchand. "It's not like you have a cast on your arm or a bandage to remind people that there's pain involved. Empathy is a difficult thing, and humans have a really difficult time empathizing with something they cannot see or have not experienced themselves." For me, this reality hit home when my husband began dealing with chronic back pain. This is a guy who is super-active and athletic. He's one of those human energy machines who do more in a day than most people do in a week. But when he started experiencing his own invisible pain issue, I had to constantly remind myself why he wasn't doing all the stuff he normally did or why he wasn't up for doing something I wanted us to do together. Or worse yet, *he* had to remind *me* that he was in pain, and when he did, I realized it had completely slipped my mind. And I'm someone who has dealt with a persistent pain issue. Once I really understood how challenging it is to empathize with an invisible health condition, I was able to bypass those feelings of resentment that would crop up during holiday visits. But I'd like to stress that understanding that empathizing with those with a persistent pain condition isn't always easy, doesn't mean you shouldn't expect any to come your way. "It's reasonable to expect empathy from the people in your life, but we sometimes have an idea what a supportive response is, and when people don't respond in those exact ways, but their intentions are good, we feel hurt and resentful. Instead of going down that road, it helps to try to understand what their intentions are, and give them a chance to respond in a better way later. Also, it's worth keeping in mind that it's hard to see someone you love in pain. To be in a situation where you're powerless to make their pain go away. We want the people we love to be well and happy. For their sake, and frankly, for ours too. We want them to feel good, so we ourselves don't have to feel bad, so we don't have to feel guilty, or worry, or take care of them, or any of that. It's human nature."

Another strategy that helped me to get past my anxiety around the holidays was learning to be okay with setting boundaries. For example, I stopped saying yes to every activity on the agenda. Or if it was still early in the evening but I was ready to leave a party or get-together, I learned to not give in to entreaties to "stay a little longer." It became easier to set these boundaries when I realized doing so actually made me a team player. "Think about why you're trying to be accommodating during the holidays," said Dr. Marchand. "Usually it's so that the people in your lives will feel good and have a positive experience. If you are comfortable and having a good experience, chances are greater that those around you will too. So it really is in everyone's best interest for you to feel good and happy. It allows you to be the best host/guest and gives you the best possible outcome."[1]

But what about the people in your life who are just never going to get it no matter what? Like Aunt Edna or Cousin Eddie who complain about you leaving the party early or hassle you for your lousy Christmas shopping efforts (gift cards for everyone!). To deal with these situations, what I do is envision myself in a bubble where I can observe that person's reaction and my reaction, but there is some distance. They don't get to get into my bubble. And from there I sort of narrate the process, like Aunt So-and-So is being rude again, now she's frowning, now she's complaining about me in some way. Narrating the process places me at an observational distance from the situation. And from there, I don't feel that I have to either fix it or control it.

Appendix A

PELVIC PAIN RESOURCES

BOOKS

Explain Pain by David Butler (NOI Group, 2nd edition, 2013)

Explain Pain resources aim to give clinicians and people in pain the power to challenge pain and to consider new models for viewing what happens during pain.

The Pain Chronicles by Melanie Thernstrom (Farrar, Straus and Giroux, 1st edition, 2010)

In *The Pain Chronicles*, Melanie Thernstrom traces conceptions of pain throughout the ages—from ancient Babylonian pain-banishing spells to modern brain imaging—to reveal the elusive, mysterious nature of pain itself.

The Anxiety and Phobia Workbook by Edmund J. Bourne (New Harbinger Publications, 4th edition, 2005)

Exercises and worksheets to overcome problems with anxiety and phobic disorders.

The Trigger Point Therapy Workbook: Your Self-Treatment Guide by Clair Davies (New Harbinger Publications, 2nd edition, 2004)

Clair Davies creates a highly effective form of pain therapy that anyone can learn. This book is a valuable contribution to the field of self-applied therapeutic bodywork.

Painful Yarns by Lorimer Moseley (Orthopedic Physical Therapy Products, 1st edition, 2007)

A collection of stories that provides an entertaining and informative way to understand modern pain biology.

Stop Endometriosis and Pelvic Pain by Andrew Cook (Femsana Press, 1st edition, 2012)

"I'm writing this book for women who have endometriosis, to help you realize you're not alone, and, above all, to offer hope." —Dr. Andrew Cook

Wild Creative (Atria Books/Beyond Words, 2014)

Through stories, visualizations, and other creative exercises, *Wild Creative* reveals groundbreaking tools for realigning the creative field and actively designing your life.

The Better Bladder Book by Wendy Cohan (Hunter House, 2010)

Wendy Cohan, RN, empowers readers to master effective self-help tools such as stress reduction, pelvic floor relaxation, and herbal remedies to conquer bladder symptoms and pelvic pain.

Healing Painful Sex by Deborah Coady (Seal Press, 2011)

Both Deborah Coady's (MD) medical expertise and Nancy Fish's (MSW, MPH) personal experience with sexual pain and her extensive professional experience as a psychotherapist provide readers with an all-inclusive understanding of the medical causes of these complex conditions as well as multidimensional medical and psychological treatments.

Secret Suffering by Susan Bilheimer and Robert J. Echenberg (2010)

Secret Suffering is the first book to open the floodgates to expose the issue of chronic sexual pain, which tears couples apart and destroys both partners' quality of life, and present in-depth interviews of suffering couples.

Heal Pelvic Pain by Amy Stein (McGraw-Hill Education, 1st edition, 2008)

Discusses stretching, toning, and relaxation exercises for pelvic pain, plus healing massages and a specialized nutrition plan for men, women, and children of all ages.

Healing Pelvic Pain and Abdominal Pain by Amy Stein

A DVD that tackles pelvic and abdominal pain, including IC/PBS, IBS, vulvodynia, endometriosis, nonbacterial prostatitis, and unexplained back, pelvic, tailbone, abdominal, bladder, bowel, genital, and sexual pain and dysfunction.

A Headache in the Pelvis by David Wise and Rodney Anderson (National Center for Pelvic Pain, 6th revised edition, 2012)

A Headache in the Pelvis adds new research recently published in the *Journal of Urology* done by the Wise-Anderson team describing the relationship of painful trigger points that refer and re-create specific symptoms of pelvic pain.

When Sex Hurts by Andrew Goldstein, Caroline Pukall, and Irwin Goldstein (Da Capo Lifelong Books, 2011)

Director of the Centers for Vulvovaginal Disorders Dr. Andrew Goldstein and leading researcher Dr. Caroline Pukall tackle the stereotypes, myths, and realities of dyspareunia, addressing its more than 20 different causes and offering the most up-to-date research. This book provides the long-awaited answers to so many women's questions.

PRODUCTS

Dilators (https://www.vaginismus.com/products/dilator_set)

Simply better products, these medical-grade dilators are smooth and comfortable, easy to control, lightweight, and safe.

Vmagic (http://www.vmagicnow.com/)

Vmagic skin cream is a 100% natural and organic solution for vulvar discomfort from irritation, dryness, and inflammation.

Pelvic Therapy Hot/Cold Pad (http://pelvicpainsolutions.com/cart/index.php?main_page=index&cPath=355)

Targets the abdomen, hips, pubic bone, pelvic floor/crotch, tailbone, and low back simultaneously with natural hot/cold therapy.

LifeStyles® SKYN® Intense Feel (http://www.lifestyles.com/category/condoms/)

SKYN is the first premium condom made from polyisoprene—a scientifically formulated non-latex material that delivers the ultimate sensitivity that is the closest thing to wearing nothing.

Restore Pressure Point Massager (http://www.gaiam.com/ product/restore-pressure-point-massager/05-58255.html)

Target pressure points, increase circulation, and alleviate sore muscles with this convenient massager. Includes a downloadable massage guide to rejuvenate tired and sore muscles throughout your body.

MuTu System (http://mutusystem.com/download-the-mutu-system-coaching-programme.html)

The complete body makeover for every mom who wants to lose the baby belly, improve pelvic floor function, and strengthen her core to get strong, fit, and body confident.

Pelvic Floor Relaxation CD for Pelvic Pain (https:// www.pelvicexercises.com.au/pelvic-exercise-products/)

Thirty minutes of guided pelvic floor muscle and whole body relaxation with breathing exercises, in two versions for men and women.

GoCommandos (http://www.gocommandos.com/)

GoCommandos all-cotton patches stick securely in your pants and jeans, eliminating conventional underwear. Now worn by many women suffering from pelvic pain and vulvar and bladder conditions who claim they are extremely soothing and comfortable.

Slippery Stuff (http://www.cmtmedical.com/ index.php?main_page=product_info&products_id=473)

Slippery Stuff is a hygienic, water-based and water-soluble, odorless, long-lasting, and latex-compatible product and is formulated to match the body's own natural lubrication.

Kolorex Intimate Care Cream (http:// www.swansonvitamins.com/natures-sources-kolorex-intimate-care-cream-1-76-oz-cream)

Soothing herbal cream free from synthetic preservatives, mineral oils, synthetic fragrances, and parabens.

Gabrialla Abdominal Binder (http://www.itamed.com/ Abdominal-Binders.html)

Decreases pressure and provides excellent support to the abdomen, waist, and lumbosacral areas.

DVD: *The Pelvic Floor Piston: Foundation for Fitness* (https:// www.juliewiebept.com/products/)

Physical therapist Julie Wiebe guides you step-by-step through new concepts, exercises, movement strategies, and body awareness tips easily integrated into your day.

DVD: *Your Pace Yoga "Relieve Pelvic Pain"* by Dustienne Miller

This DVD was created by Dustienne Miller, a board-certified women's health physical therapist and Kripalu yoga teacher. This yoga home program was specifically designed for men and women who are healing chronic pelvic pain. The DVD weaves together breath work, meditation, body awareness, and gentle yoga postures. This stress-relieving program can be practiced in as little as 20 minutes, making it possible to fit into daily life.

TheraWand (http://www.therawand.com)

TheraWand has been found by physical therapists to be indispensable in pelvic floor treatments, including but not limited to trigger point (myofascial) release, painful intercourse, scar tissue, sensitivity, tight vaginal opening, vaginismus, anorgasmia, prostate massage, and more.

Reduce Sexual Pain Guides **(http://sexualrehab.com/Additional-Resources.html)**

PDF guides that provide a new way to look at sex for couples, as well as more information on pleasurable products, and activities.

Cushions

Cushion Your Assets (http://www.cushionyourassets.com/)
TheraSeat (http://www.cmtmedical.com/in-dex.php?main_page=product_info&products_id=415)
WonderGel Cushion (http://www.bedbathandbeyond.com/1/1/197992-wondergel-extreme-seat-cushion.html)

BLOGS/VIDEOS

Dr. Jen Gunter, https://drjengunter.wordpress.com/
Julie Wiebe, PT, https://www.juliewiebept.com/blog/
Blog About Pelvic Pain, http://www.blogaboutpelvicpain.com/
Sexual Healing
Body in Mind, http://www.bodyinmind.org/
IC Network, http://www.ic-network.com/
The Pelvic Guru, http://pelvicguru.com/
Understanding Pain: What to do about it in less than five minutes? https://www.youtube.com/watch?v=4b8oB757DKc&feature=player_embedded
Pain Management Meditation Video, https://www.youtube.com/watch?v=2kVKx-6uzsE
Pelvic Floor Part 1—The Pelvic Diaphragm—3D Anatomy Video Tutorial, http://anatomyzone.com/tutorials/musculoskeletal/pelvic-floor/
Pelvic Floor Part 2—Perineal Membrane and Deep Perineal Pouch, https://www.youtube.com/watch?v=q0Ax3rLFc6M

SUPPORT GROUPS

Happy Pelvis, https://groups.yahoo.com/neo/groups/happypelvis/info
Pelvic Pain Support Network, https://healthunlocked.com/pelvicpain
Endometriosis Groups, http://endometriosis.org/support/support-
    groups/
Baby Center, http://community.babycenter.com/
Golden Gate Mothers Group, http://www.ggmg.org/
IC Network, http://www.ic-network.com/forum/forum.php
Pelvic Organ Prolapse Support, http://
    www.pelvicorganprolapsesupport.org/
Women's Health Foundation, http://womenshealthfoundation.org/

Appendix B

EVALUATION INTERVIEW: COMPLETE LIST OF QUESTIONS

SYMPTOMS INFORMATION:

- What do you think caused your symptoms?
- When did your symptoms begin?
- Describe the quality of the symptoms—itching, burning, aching, etc.
- What makes your symptoms worse?
- What makes your symptoms better?
- Are your symptoms intermittent or constant?

URINARY INFORMATION:

- Do you have difficulty initiating your urinary stream?
- Is the stream weak or interrupted?
- How many times per day do you void?
- How many times per night do you void?
- Do certain foods, beverages, positions, or activities change your urinary function?
- Do you experience pain or burning before, during, or after voiding? If so, where?
- Do you leak urine when you cough, sneeze, or laugh?
- Do you leak urine when you feel the urge to void?
- Do you leak urine without realizing it?

BOWEL INFORMATION:

- Do you have a history of constipation and/or IBS? If yes, is it currently controlled?
- How often do you have a bowel movement?
- Do you have a history of anal fissures or hemorrhoids?
- Do you experience pain or burning before, during, or after a bowel movement?
- Do you have difficulty evacuating stool?
- Has the shape or quality of your bowel movements changed recently?

SEXUAL AND GENITAL INFORMATION:

Men:

- Are you able to obtain an erection?
- Are you able to ejaculate?
- Do you experience pain before, during, or after ejaculation?
- Have you noticed a change in the quality of your erection and/or ejaculate?
- Do you have genital or pelvic itching?

Women:

- Do you experience pain with penetration?
- Do you experience pain with deep thrusting or certain positions?
- Do you have painful menses?
- Are you able to achieve an orgasm?
- Do you have pain before, during, or after intercourse and/or orgasm?
- Do you experience genital or pelvic itching?
- Do you have a history of urinary tract infections?
- Do you have a history of yeast infections?
- Do you feel the presence of a foreign body in the vagina or as if things are falling out of the vagina?

NOTES

FOREWORD

1. There is some debate regarding the use of the terminology "persistent pelvic pain" or "chronic pelvic pain." Currently, the thinking is that pelvic pain is not always chronic, that in many cases it can be cured or at least very well controlled. Thus, "chronic" is thought by many experts to be an inappropriate name and "persistent" more appropriate to the condition.

INTRODUCTION

1. T Jackson et al., "The Impact of Threatening Information about Pain on Coping and Pain Tolerance," *British Journal of Health Psychology* 10 (2005): 441–451.

1. PELVIC PAIN 101

1. R Fillingim et al., "The ACTTION-American Pain Society Pain Taxonomy (AAPT): An Evidence-Based and Multidimensional Approach to Classifying Chronic Pain Conditions," *Journal of Pain* 15, no. 3 (March 2014): 241–249.

2. HOW DID I GET PELVIC PAIN? THE IMPORTANCE OF UNCOVERING CONTRIBUTING FACTORS

1. I Goldstein and L Burrows, "Can Oral Contraceptives Cause Vestibulo-dynia?" *Journal of Sexual Medicine* 7 (2010): 1585–1587.

3. DEMYSTIFYING THE NEUROMUSCULAR IMPAIRMENTS THAT CAUSE PELVIC PAIN

1. D Simons et al., *Travell and Simons' Myofascial Pain and Dysfunction: The Trigger Point Manual* (LLW, 1998).

6. GUIDE TO NAVIGATING TREATMENT OPTIONS

1. RM Moldwin and JY Fariello, "Myofascial Trigger Points of the Pelvic Floor: Associations with Urological Pain Syndromes and Treatment Strategies Including Injection Therapy," *Current Urology Report* 14, no. 5 (October 2013): 409–417.

2. *Ibid.*

3. SH Richeimer et al., "Utilization Patterns of Tricyclic Antidepressants in a Multidisciplinary Pain Clinic: A Survey," *Clinical Journal of Pain* 13 (1997): 324–329.

4. A Beydoun et al., "Gabapentin: Pharmacokinetics, Efficacy, and Safety," *Clinical Neuropharmacology* 14 (1995): 469–481.

5. DJ Hewitt, "The Use of NMDA-Receptor Antagonists in the Treatment of Chronic Pain," *Clinical Journal of Pain* 16, no. 2 (2000): S73–S79.

6. D Engeler et al., "General Treatment of Chronic Pelvic Pain: Guidelines on Chronic Pelvic Pain," European Association of Urology (February 2012): 122–130.

7. P Gupta et al., "Percutaneous Tibial Nerve Stimulation and Sacral Neuromodulation: An Update," *Current Urology Report* 16, no. 2 (February 2015): 4.

8. KM Alo and J Holsheimer, "New Trends in Neuromodulation for the Management of Neuropathic Pain," *Neurosurgery* 50 (2002): 690–703.

9. D Byrd and S Mackey, "Pulsed Radio Frequency for Chronic Pain," *Current Pain and Headaches Report* 1 (January 12, 2008): 37–41.

10. CL Swanson et al., "Localized Provoked Vestibulodynia: Outcomes after Modified Vestibulectomy," *Journal of Reproductive Medicine* 59, no. 3–4 (March–April 2014): 121–126.

11. JM Danford et al., "Postoperative Pain Outcomes after Transvaginal Mesh Revision," *International Urogynecology Journal* 26, no. 1 (January 2015): 65–69.

7. THE PELVIC FLOOR AND PREGNANCY: TREATING NEW MOMS RIGHT

1. M Beckmann and O Stock, "Antenatal Perineal Massage for Reducing Perineal Trauma," *Cochrane Database of Systemic Reviews* 4 (2013).

2. WH Wu et al., "Pregnancy Related Pelvic Girdle Pain: Terminology, Clinical Presentation, and Prevalence," *European Spine Journal* 13 (2004): 575–589.

3. K Bo, "Evaluation of Female Pelvic Floor Muscle Function and Strength," *Physical Therapy* 85 (2005): 269–282.

4. JS Boissonnault and MJ Blaschak, "Incidence of Diastasis Recti Abdominis during the Childbearing Years," *Physical Therapy Journal* 68 (1988): 1082–1086.

5. J Martin et al., "Births: Final Data for 2013," *Centers for Disease Control and Prevention National Vital Statistics Reports* 64 (2015).

6. K Bo, "Evaluation of Female Pelvic Floor Muscle Function and Strength," *Physical Therapy Journal* 85 (2005): 269–282.

7. Sara Fox, e-mail message to author, February 14, 2015.

8. Mark Conway, e-mail message to author, February 16, 2015.

8. PELVIC PAIN AND SEX: THE FACTS

1. L Pink, V Rancourt, and A Gordon, "Persistent Genital Arousal in Women with Pelvic and Genital Pain," *Journal of Obstetrics and Gynaecology Canada* 36, no. 4 (April 2014): 324–330.

2. Heather Howard, Ph.D. (board certified sexologist) in discussion with the author, March 6, 2015.

3. *Ibid.*

4. Erica Marchand, Ph.D. (psychologist specializing in couples and sex therapy) in discussion with the author, March 3, 2015.

5. Rose Hartzell, Ph.D. (certified sex educator and therapist) in discussion with the author, March 11, 2015.

6. Marchand, March 3, 2015.

7. Howard, March 6, 2015.

8. Hartzell, March 11, 2015.

9. Howard, March 6, 2015.

12. TIPS FOR DAY-TO-DAY LIVING

1. Dr. Erica Marchand, Ph.D. (licensed psychologist), in discussion with the author, November 15, 2014.

BIBLIOGRAPHY

Alo, KM and J Holsheimer. "New Trends in Neuromodulation for the Management of Neuropathic Pain." *Neurosurgery* 50 (2002): 690–703.

Apte, G et al. "Chronic Female Pelvic Pain: Part I: Clinical Pathoanatomy and Examination of the Pelvic Region." *Pain Practice* 12 (2012): 88–110.

Beckmann, M and O Stock. "Antenatal Perineal Massage for Reducing Perineal Trauma." *Cochrane Database of Systemic Reviews* 4 (2013).

Bergman, J and S Zeitlin. "Prostatitis and Chronic Prostatitis/Chronic Pelvic Pain Syndrome." *Expert Review of Neurotherapeutics* 7 (2007): 301–307.

Beydoun, A et al. "Gabapentin: Pharmacokinetics, Efficacy, and Safety." *Clinical Neuropharmacology* 14 (1995): 469–481.

Bo, K. "Evaluation of Female Pelvic Floor Muscle Function and Strength." *Physical Therapy Journal* 85 (2005): 269–282.

Boissonnault, JS and MJ Blaschak. "Incidence of Diastasis Recti Abdominis during the Childbearing Years." *Physical Therapy Journal* 68 (1988): 1082–1086.

Byrd, D and S Mackey. "Pulsed Radio Frequency for Chronic Pain." *Current Pain and Headaches Report* 1 (January 12, 2008): 37–41.

Danford, JM, DJ Osborn, WS Reynolds, DH Biller, and RR Dmochowski. "Postoperative Pain Outcomes after Transvaginal Mesh Revision." *International Urogynecology Journal* 26, no. 1 (January 2015): 65–69.

Engeler, D, AP Baranowski, S Elneil, J Hughes, EJ Messelink, P Oliveira, A van Ophoven, and AC de C Williams. "General Treatment of Chronic Pelvic Pain: Guidelines on Chronic Pelvic Pain." European Association of Urology (February 2012): 122–130.

Fillingim, R, S Bruehl, and R Dworkin et al. "The ACTTION-American Pain Society Pain Taxonomy (AAPT): An Evidence-Based and Multidimensional Approach to Classifying Chronic Pain Conditions." *Journal of Pain* 15, no. 3 (March 2014): 241–249.

Goldstein, I and L Burrows. "Can Oral Contraceptives cause Vestibulodynia?" *Journal of Sexual Medicine* 7 (2010): 1585–1587.

Gupta, P, MJ Ehlert, LT Sirls, and KM Peters. "Percutaneous Tibial Nerve Stimulation and Sacral Neuromodulation: An Update." *Current Urology Report* 16, no. 2 (February 2015): 4.

Gyang et al. "Musculoskeletal Causes of Chronic Pelvic Pain: What Every Gynecologist Should Know." *American College of Obstetrics and Gynecology* 121 (2013): 645–650.

Habermacher, G, J Chason, and A Schaeffer. "Chronic Prostatitis/Chronic Pelvic Pain Syndrome." *Annual Review of Medicine* 57 (2006): 195–206.

Hewitt, DJ. "The Use of NMDA-Receptor Antagonists in the Treatment of Chronic Pain." *Clinical Journal of Pain* 16, no. 2 (2000): S73–S79.

Jackson, T, L Pope, T Nagasaka, A Fritch, T Iezzi, and H Chen. "The Impact of Threatening Information about Pain on Coping and Pain Tolerance." *British Journal of Health Psychology* 10 (2005): 441–451.

Jones, MD, J Booth, JL Taylor, and BK Barry. "Aerobic Training Increases Pain Tolerance in Healthy Individuals." *Medicine & Science in Sports & Exercise* 46 (2014): 1640–1647.

Martin, J, B Hamilton, M Osterman, S Curtin, and T Mathews. "Births: Final Data for 2013." *Centers for Disease Control and Prevention National Vital Statistics Reports* 64 (2015).

McDonald, EA, D Gartland, R Small, and SJ Brown. "Dyspareunia and Childbirth: A Prospective Cohort Study." *British Journal of Obstetrics and Gynecology* 21 January 2015, doi: 10.1111/1471-0528.13263.

Moldwin, RM and JY Fariello. "Myofascial Trigger Points of the Pelvic Floor: Associations with Urological Pain Syndromes and Treatment Strategies Including Injection Therapy." *Current Urology Report* 14, no. 5 (October 2013): 409–417.

Pink, L, V Rancourt, and A Gordon. "Persistent Genital Arousal in Women with Pelvic and Genital Pain." *Journal of Obstetrics and Gynaecology Canada* 36, no. 4 (April 2014): 324–330.

Richeimer, SH et al. "Utilization Patterns of Tricyclic Antidepressants in a Multidisciplinary Pain Clinic: A Survey." *Clinical Journal of Pain* 13 (1997): 324–329.

Sadownik, LA. "Etiology, Diagnosis, and Clinical Management of Vulvodynia." *International Journal of Women's Health* 6 (2014): 437–449.

Schwertner-Tiepelmann, N, R Thakar, AH Sultan, and R Tunn. "Obstetric Levator Ani Muscle Injuries: Current Status." *Ultrasound Obstetrics and Gynecology* 39 (2012): 372–383.

Simons, D, J Travell, L Simons, and B Cummings. *Travell and Simons' Myofascial Pain and Dysfunction: The Trigger Point Manual.* (LLW, 1998).

Swanson, CL, JA Rueter, JE Olson, AL Weaver, and CR Stanhope. "Localized Provoked Vestibulodynia: Outcomes after Modified Vestibulectomy." *Journal of Reproductive Medicine* 59, no. 3–4 (March–April 2014): 121–126.

Vleeming, A, HB Albert, and HC Ostgaard et al. "European Guidelines for the Diagnosis and Treatment of Pelvic Girdle Pain." *European Spine Journal* 17 (2008): 794–819.

Wu, WH, OG Meijer, K Uegaki, JM Mens, JH van Dieen, PI Wuisman, and HC Ostgaard. "Pregnancy Related Pelvic Girdle Pain: Terminology, Clinical Presentation, and Prevalence." *European Spine Journal* 13 (2004): 575–589.

Zondervan, KT, PL Yudkin, MP Vessey, MG Dawes, DH Barlow, and SH Kennedy. "Prevalence and Incidence of Chronic Pelvic Pain in Primary Care: Evidence from a National General Practice Database." *Journal of Obstetrics and Gynecology* 106 (1999): 1149–1155.

INDEX

acupuncture.. *See* alternative medicine

alternative medicine, 99–100

American Physical Therapy Association, 55

biomechanical abnormalities, 25, 68

biopsychosocial treatment approach, 10

botulinum toxin type A injections, 87–88

central nervous system, 44, 45, 76–77, 95–96

central sensitization, 44, 45, 76–77, 95–96, 97

cesarean section scar. *See* scar tissue

chronic nonbacterial prostatitis, 80

chronic pelvic pain syndrome. *See* chronic nonbacterial prostatitis

cluneal nerve, 45

coccygodynia. *See* tailbone pain

cognitive behavioral therapy, 96

constipation, 24

cushions, 183

diagnostic testing, 99

diastasis rectus abdominis, 109, 110, 111, 205n2; correction of, 114–115; evaluation of, 113; precautions, 113–114; prevalence, 112; prevention, 112; symptoms, 111–112

dry needling, 86

dyspareunia, 72

endometriosis, 27, 29

erectile dysfunction. *See* sexual dysfunction

exercise, 157–163, 164

fibromyalgia, 29

finding a doctor, 53–54

finding a physical therapist, 55

fissures, 25

footwear, 185

genitofemoral nerve, 44, 45

Happy Pelvis, 56

Herman and Wallace Pelvic Rehabilitation Institute, 56

hormones, 27

iliohypogastric nerve, 45

ilioinguinal nerve, 42, 44, 45

impairments, 33; biomechanical, 25, 68; connective tissue, 41, 66, 67; myofascial trigger points, 37–40, 39, 40, 66; muscular, 34–35; neurodynamics, 42, 68; neuromuscular, 11

incontinence, 117

infection, 21–22

intercourse. *See* sex

interdisciplinary treatment approach, 10, 75; communicating with providers,

ABOUT THE AUTHORS

Stephanie Prendergast and **Elizabeth Rummer** are the founders of the Pelvic Health and Rehabilitation Center (PHRC), a physical therapy practice that focuses solely on the treatment of pelvic pain/dysfunction for men and women. With four locations in California (Los Angeles, San Francisco, Berkeley, and Los Gatos) and one East Coast location in Waltham, Massachusetts, PHRC is the premier pelvic floor rehabilitation clinic in the country. Stephanie and Liz are well-recognized experts and thought leaders in the treatment of pelvic pain/dysfunction. They lecture worldwide and have been interviewed by and/or contributed articles to publications such as the *New York Times* and the *Los Angeles Times* along with several medical textbooks, including *Chronic Pelvic Pain and Dysfunction: Practical Physical Medicine; Abdominal and Pelvic Pain: From Definition to Best Practice;* and *Fascia: The Tensional Network of the Human Body.* In addition, they hold leadership roles in numerous pelvic pain–related organizations. Stephanie was the first physical therapist to be elected as president of the International Pelvic Pain Society in 2013 after serving on their board of directors for 10 years. They are also involved in the Global Society for Endometriosis and Pelvic Pain Surgeons, and Stephanie was a cofounder, lecturer, and scientific program chair for the World Congress on Abdominal and Pelvic Pain in Amsterdam in 2013, in Nice in 2015, and in Washington, DC, in 2017.